# Primary Child and Adolescent Mental Health

# Primary Child and Adolescent Mental Health

A practical guide
## VOLUME II
Second Edition

### Dr Quentin Spender

*Consultant in Child and Adolescent Psychiatry*
*Wolverhampton City Primary Care Trust*
*Wolverhampton, UK*

### Dr Judith Barnsley

*Consultant in Child and Adolescent Psychiatry*
*Dorset Healthcare University NHS Foundation Trust*
*Poole, UK*

### Alison Davies

*Primary Mental Health Worker*
*Sussex Partnership NHS Foundation Trust*
*Chichester, UK*

and

### Dr Jenny Murphy

*Clinical Psychologist*
*Dorset Healthcare University NHS Foundation Trust*
*Poole, UK*

Radcliffe Publishing
London • New York

**Radcliffe Publishing Ltd**
33–41 Dallington Street
London
EC1V 0BB
United Kingdom

**www.radcliffepublishing.com**

Electronic catalogue and worldwide online ordering facility.

First Edition 2001

British Library Cataloguing in Publication Data

A catalogue record for this book is available from the British Library.

ISBN-13: 978 184619 314 9 (box set)
ISBN-13: 978 184619 543 3 (volume II)

Typeset by KnowledgeWorks Global Ltd, Chennai, India
Printed and bound by Cadmus Communications, USA

# Contents

# Preface to the second edition

In the decade since the first edition of this book, the way in which mental health services in the United Kingdom are provided to children and adolescents has changed in a number of ways. Although geographical uniformity has proved difficult to achieve, frontline services have been extensively developed to improve the mental health of the under-18 population.

The aim of this book is to give those working at the frontline – the first professionals that a child or parent may meet when asking for help – a practical guide about what to do. The chapters are structured to enable relevant theoretical issues to be summarised simply, followed by detailed suggestions about how to gather relevant information and how to help, leaving referral to specialised services as a last resort.

Our vision is that a whole variety of professionals to whom children or parents may turn for help will have at their fingertips a means of understanding the problems presented, and will be able to offer straightforward ways of helping. Professionals at the frontline need training and advice from more experienced and highly trained colleagues; but we hope this book will also play a role in their professional development and provide an additional source of support, either as a component of learning or as a resource for teaching.

It would be foolhardy not to acknowledge some of the difficulties inherent in providing a universal Child and Adolescent Mental Health Service (CAMHS) that can meet everyone's needs. These barriers include the following.

➤ *Agency cooperation* – Using the broadest definition of CAMHS, services are provided and professionals employed by not only the National Health Service but also by Educational and Social Care organisations; others play a role, such as the youth criminal justice system, substance misuse services and counselling charities. A single child may have contact with a bewildering array of different organisations and individuals, making effective cooperation between them a significant challenge.

➤ *Management issues* – The joint management of Education and Social Care, and the appointment of jointly funded Commissioners, has been introduced to help coordinate the main involved agencies. There remains tremendous variation in management structures. Considering now the narrow definition of CAMHS, specialised services may be part of Mental Health Trusts, Primary Care Trusts or Trusts providing hospital paediatric care. Within these Trusts, specialised CAMHS may be in a directorate with a variety of bedfellows, for instance: adult mental health; adult learning difficulty; community paediatrics; hospital paediatrics; health visiting; school nursing; and many others. Some Trusts favour medics in managerial roles such as that of CAMHS Clinical Director; some Trusts prefer non-clinicians for service management roles; others prefer clinicians such as nurses, psychologists or social workers for both clinical and service management roles.

➤ This variation in management structures is part of the *'postcode lottery'*, meaning that services may be available in one area but not another, and that *where* the child and family live may be as much a factor in determining what help is available as the skill-mix of professionals. Another component of this is that areas of deprivation have higher per capita funding, but in relatively affluent areas, a higher proportion of the population in need may present for help, with the result that services may paradoxically be more stretched in more affluent areas. This can be exacerbated by the cost of housing contributing to difficulties in recruiting staff. The independent sector is just as patchy in its provision (perhaps more). Added to all this is the variation in the four countries of the UK: England, Scotland, Wales and Northern Ireland. We have not attempted in this book to do justice to this, but have stuck to what we know, which is our own practice within three different regions of England: we cannot claim with our limited joint experience to understand the range of service provision within even *one* country.

➤ *Service lacunae* (gaps in what is provided) have persisted, despite a variety of attempts to make services more uniform, such as the National Service Framework[1] and the establishment of a peer-reviewing system.[2] An example is the service received by children with learning difficulties and their families, which is still extremely patchy and highly variable.

➤ *Funding issues* – It is beyond the scope of this book to present the arguments about the inequitable share of the funding cake allocated to under-18s compared to other age groups, or mental health problems compared to other categories of ill health. Killers such as cancer, heart disease or premature birth are more likely to get the sort of publicity that mobilises political will. Some have described CAMHS as the 'Cinderella of Cinderellas'. Periods of investment tend to be followed by periods of renewed financial stringency. Joint commissioning arrangements may not be able to prevent huge sums being spent on highly specialised provision for a small number of individuals, thus stifling investment in small-scale outpatient teams: a larger scale preventative approach may be necessary for this.

➤ *Customer confusion* – All of this variation may leave parents very confused about how best to access help for their child. Professionals may also be confused about who is best placed to deliver the best help at the best time: the professional who first sees the child may be chosen more by accident than by any logical process. Some acronyms (abbreviations) may add to the overall confusion. We give here a selection:

| | | |
|---|---|---|
| — | ABE | Achieving Best Evidence |
| — | ASBO | Antisocial Behaviour Order |
| — | ASSIST | Asylum Seeker Support Initiative Short Term |
| — | BESD | Behavioural, Educational and Social Difficulties |
| — | BEST | Behavioural and Educational Support Team |
| — | BOSS | Business Opportunity Sourcing Service |
| — | BPD | Borderline Personality Disorder |
| — | BPD | Bipolar Disorder |
| — | BPD | Broncho-Pulmonary Dysplasia |
| — | BPS | British Psychological Society |
| — | CAF | Common Assessment Framework |
| — | CAFE | Child and Adolescent Faculty Executive |
| — | CAP | Child and Adolescent Psychiatry |
| — | CORC | CAMHS Outcome Research Consortium |
| — | CPD | Continuing Professional Development |
| — | CPD | Continuous Peritoneal Dialysis |
| — | CPS | Crown Prosecution Service |
| — | CRB | Criminal Records Bureau |
| — | DAT | Drug and Alcohol Team |
| — | DAT | Drug Action Team |
| — | DCSF | Department for Children, Schools and Families |
| — | DNA | Did Not Arrive |
| — | DNA | Deoxyribonucleic acid |
| — | DoH | Department of Health |
| — | DTO | Detention and Training Order |
| — | EBD | Educational and Behavioural Difficulties |
| — | EBPD | Emerging Borderline Personality Disorder |
| — | E2E | Entry to Employment |
| — | FAST | Family Advice and Support Team |
| — | FIP | Family Intervention Project |
| — | FRT | Family Resource Team |
| — | GAP | Guideline Appraisal Panel |
| — | HAVOC | Having an Alternative View of Crime |
| — | HMYOI | Her Majesty's Young Offender Institution |
| — | IRS worker | Integrated Resettlement Support worker |
| — | ISP | Initial Supervision Plan |
| — | ISSP | Intensive Supervision and Surveillance Programme |
| — | JAR | Joint Area Review |
| — | KYPE | Keeping Young People Engaged |
| — | LAC | Looked-After Children |
| — | LD | Learning Difficulty |
| — | MAPPA | Multi-Agency Public Protection Arrangements |
| — | MAST | Multi-Agency Support Team |
| — | MHPW | Mental Health and Psychological Wellbeing |
| — | MLD | Moderate Learning Difficulty |

- NEET — Not in Education, Employment or Training
- NHS — National Health Service
- NICE — National Institute for Health and Clinical Excellence
- OFSTED — Office for Standards in Education
- OoH — Out of Hours
- PAYP — Positive Activities for Young People
- PCAMHW — Primary Child and Adolescent Mental Health Worker
- PCSO — Police Community Service Officer
- PCT — Primary Care Trust
- PDP — Personal Development Plan
- PHEW — Psychological Health and Emotional Wellbeing
- PMHW — Primary Mental Health Worker
- PREMs — Patient-Reported Experience Measures
- PROMs — Patient-Reported Outcome Measures
- PRU — Pupil Referral Unit
- PTSD — Post Traumatic Stress Disorder
- PSA — Parenting Support Adviser
- PSR — Pre-Sentence Report
- RAP — Recurrent Abdominal Pain
- RAP — Resource Allocation Panel
- RAP — Resettlement and Aftercare Provision
- RoH — Risk of Harm
- SENCo — Special Educational Needs Coordinator
- SIG — Special Interest Group
- SIPS — Social Inclusion and Pupil Support
- SLA — Service Level Agreement
- SLD — Severe Learning Difficulty
- SMART — Specific, Measurable, Achievable, Realistic and Time-bounded
- SPP — Senior Parenting Practitioner
- SSIW — Social Services Inspectorate for Wales
- TAC — Team Around the Child
- TaMHS — Targeted Mental Health in Schools
- TPU — Teenage Pregnancy Unit
- VLO — Victim Liaison Officer
- WPI — Wales Programme for Improvement
- YADAS — Young Adults' Drug and Alcohol Service
- YIP — Youth Inclusion Programme
- YISP — Youth Inclusion Support Panel
- YJB — Youth Justice Board
- YOI — Young Offender's Institution
- YOIS — Youth Offending Information System
- YOT — Youth Offending Team
- ... and many others.

Another change since the first edition of this book is the increasing avail-ability of protocols and guidelines developed to reduce the risks inherent in any dabbling with other people's mental health – and the variability of clinical approach inevitable in a multidisciplinary field.  Some are local, others are national, in particular the Scottish Intercollegiate Guideline Network (SIGN)[3] guidelines in Scotland and the National Institute for Health and Clinical Excellence (NICE)[4] guidelines for the whole UK. These aim to make clinical practice more evidence-based and uniform, and should in theory reduce the postcode lottery.

Other developments such as leaflets,[5] information sheets,[6] websites[7] and chari-ties[8] have aimed at reducing the confusion for families of knowing which profes-sion they should go to when, and the confusion for professionals about whether they are duplicating others' work, or alternatively allowing families to fall into the gaps between services. Various ways of combining professionals from different disciplines into teams who are more coordinated, or more convenient for fami-lies, or more convenient for agencies, have been devised (see some of the acro-nyms above), but there seems to be a remarkable lack of uniformity. The Common Assessment Framework[9] is an attempt to save professionals in different agencies from carrying out repeated initial assessments that ask all the same questions: once done by one agency, it should be shared electronically with others who need to be involved. The use of Electronic Health Records is already common in Health Centres, and is due to spread to specialist CAMHS as we write this edition. We anticipate some difficulties including all the information gathered by specialist CAMHS in electronic form – not least because of concerns about who will access the information.

Just as the expectations placed on professionals working in all levels of CAMHS have changed in a decade, so have the lives of young people been transformed by readily available internet access. Social contact can now take place without any-one leaving their rooms. Cyber-bullying and internet grooming (leading to sexual abuse) have added new dimensions to the hazards of adolescent relationships. Whereas previously we might have worried whether we should allow a parent to show us her daughter's diary without permission, we may now be worried about whether to look at a personal blog, and how we should respond to what we may find there. Similarly, whilst there is much helpful information on the Internet, young people can also access unhelpful sites such as pro-anorexia and pro-suicide websites that compound their despair and undermine the help they may be offered or at least need.

One change that has particularly affected the target audience for this book is the advent, at least in some areas, of the Primary Child and Adolescent Mental Health Worker, variously abbreviated as PCAMHW or PMHW. This specialism was just being developed as the first edition was being published. The initial idea for the book (which we must credit to Professor Peter Hill) was as a source of practical information for those working in primary care – the case exam-ples were written with General Practitioners in mind – but GPs may have been only a small proportion of the book's readership. Professor Hill was also part of the group that developed[10] the idea of the Four Tier system and the Primary Child and Adolescent Mental Health Worker (for further details *see* Chapter 1: Context).

The first edition seems to have been devoured by a variety of professionals doing Tier 1 and Tier 2 work, and we hope this edition will cater more overtly for these groups. We have shifted the emphasis to make the book suitable for any profession to whom the Primary Child and Adolescent Mental Health Worker consults. We hope the book will enable frontline practitioners (Tier 1 or universal services) to catch child mental health conditions at an early stage so that interventions can be provided without having to wait for specialised services (Tier 3 or targeted services) to become involved. The authorship, instead of being a mixture of Child and Adolescent Psychiatrists and GPs, is now a mixture of Child and Adolescent Psychiatrists and Primary Child and Adolescent Mental Health Workers.

Rather than tinker with the first edition, we have rewritten the whole book, reorganising some of the chapter structure, but keeping the more successful chapters while updating them. We have persisted in our strategy of breaking-up the text by liberal use of bullet points, tables, case examples, summary boxes (including 'Practice Points' and 'Alarm Bells') and figures. The most striking change is perhaps the first main section of the book (Chapters 2 to 4), which emphasises our developmental approach by describing the differences between three important development stages: pre-school, middle childhood and adolescence. In particular, the chapter on middle childhood contains much of the content of the first chapter in the first edition, which was entitled 'Assessment'. We have also changed the title, to reflect the change in emphasis.

*A note on terminology:* We have alternated the female and male pronoun when talking about an unspecified child (or parent). We are aware there are various definitions of 'children' (for instance: under-13, Gillick incompetent, under-16 or under-18); 'adolescents' (12–25 being perhaps the most inclusive); and 'young people' (for instance, 16- and 17-year-olds, 11–19 or seven to 25). But we have used these terms colloquially, without attempting to stick to one definition. We have also used the terms 'parent' and 'carer' interchangeably (so as to avoid the cumbersome phrase 'parent or carer'). We have tried to keep abbreviations to a minimum, but have allowed ourselves to use a few, such as: 'CAMHS' for Child and Adolescent Mental Health Services; 'ADHD' for Attention-Deficit/Hyperactivity Disorder; GCSEs for General Certificate of Secondary Education exams; and 'DVDs' for Digital Versatile Discs.

*A note on case examples:* We have pursued a policy of peppering the text liberally with these, in order to break up the text, maintain clinical relevance and keep things interesting. The case examples vary in their origins: some are based on a single case, with enough details altered to make the identity unrecognisable to anyone but the child and family; some incorporate details of more than one case; and some are fictionalised on the basis of our clinical experience (so effectively incorporating the details of many cases).

We hope that our labours will enable our readers to improve the mental health and emotional well-being of children throughout the United Kingdom, and possibly elsewhere.

**Quentin Spender**
**Judith Barnsley**
**Alison Davies**
**Jenny Murphy**
*April 2011*

## REFERENCES

1 www.dh.gov.uk/en/Publicationsandstatistics/Publications/PublicationsPolicyAnd Guidance/DH_4089114
2 www.rcpsych.ac.uk/crtu/centreforqualityimprovement/qinmaccamhs.aspx
3 www.sign.ac.uk
4 www.nice.org.uk
5 www.rcpsych.ac.uk
6 CAMHS Evidence Based Practice Unit. *Choosing What's Best For You: what scientists have found helps children and young people who are sad, worried or troubled.* London: CAMHS publications; July 2007. Available at: www.annafreud.org/ebpu (accessed 20 March 2011).
7 www.mentalhealth.org.uk
8 www.youngminds.org.uk
9 www.education.gov.uk/childrenandyoungpeople/strategy/integratedworking/caf/a0068957/the-caf-process
10 Health Advisory Service. *Together We Stand: the commissioning, role and management of child and adolescent mental health services.* London: HMSO; 1995.

# About the authors

**Dr Quentin Spender**, Consultant in Child and Adolescent Psychiatry, Wolverhampton City Primary Care Trust, Wolverhampton, UK

**Dr Judith Barnsley**, Consultant in Child and Adolescent Psychiatry, Dorset Healthcare University NHS Foundation Trust, Poole, UK

**Alison Davies**, Primary Mental Health Worker, Sussex Partnership NHS Foundation Trust, Chichester, UK

**Dr Jenny Murphy**, Clinical Psychologist, Dorset Healthcare University NHS Foundation Trust, Poole, UK

# Acknowledgements

This book germinated from an idea that we must credit to Professor Emeritus Peter Hill, who wanted to fashion a companion volume to the same publisher's *The Child Surveillance Handbook*,[1] of which he was an initial co-author. Along with our own changing co-authorship, we have benefited from the direct or indirect input of the following: Rosemarie Berry, Chrissy Boardman, Teri Boutwood, Nina Bunce, Anna Calver, Esther Crawley, David Candy, Steve Clarke, David Rex, Moira Doolan, Danya Glaser, Gill Goodwillie, Sue Horobin, Amelia Kerswell, Karen King, Sebastian Kraemer, Karen Majors, Rebecca Park, Joanna Pearse, Nigel Speight, Anne Stewart and Wendy Woodhouse. We would also like to thank the children and families whom we have all seen in our clinical work: they have taught us so much, and many of them have provided us with the stories for our case examples.

## Note

1 First edition published in 1990, second edition published in 1994 and third edition published in 2009. Hall D, Williams J, Elliman D. *The Child Surveillance Handbook*. 3rd ed. London and New York: Radcliffe Publishing; 2009.

# PART 3

# Preschool

# CHAPTER 14

# Postnatal depression

## INTRODUCTION

There is a substantial psychiatric morbidity associated with childbirth. At least 10% of women will have a major depressive episode in the year following childbirth. The risk is higher in the first three months than the following nine months.[1] The subject is included in this book because of the well-established effects of postnatal depression on early mother/child interactions and on children's cognitive and social development.

In the postnatal period, a woman is at greater risk than at any other time in her life of suffering from a severe depressive illness, becoming psychotic, being referred to a psychiatrist, and of being admitted to a psychiatric hospital. Untreated postnatal depression has a number of effects upon the mother including difficulties with close relationships, social isolation, and in 30% of mothers it continues into the second year of the child's life.

Depressed mothers are less sensitive, less attentive and more critical of their infants.[2] The effects of untreated postnatal depression on children, compared to a control group whose mothers are not depressed, may include:
➤ impaired cognitive development[3]
➤ less warmth and positive interaction between child and parent (both ways)
➤ the development of an insecure attachment, usually of the avoidant type
➤ behavioural difficulties[4]
➤ poor growth.[5]

### Causal theories

There is as yet no agreement about a hormonal basis for postnatal depression, although genetic studies suggest that biological factors must be relevant. Obstetric complications may increase risk, but possibly only in those with a previous history of depressive disorder. A psychiatric history, particularly of depressive disorder, raises the risk – especially if the previous depression occurred within a year of childbirth. Social factors have been shown to increase the risk, including: an unplanned pregnancy; recent stressful life events; unemployment in either the mother or father; not breast-feeding; marital conflict; and lack of personal support from spouse, family and friends.[6] It seems that some women may suffer from specific triggering of a mood disorder by childbirth.[7] Childbirth is a major life event linked with many expectations that can lead to disappointment. Both partners have to adjust to the new baby and changes in their relationship. Difficulties in making this adjustment may reveal cracks that were previously concealed. The nuclear family can make it very easy to become isolated after childbirth. Factors in the child are also important: an irritable baby (who is hard to handle), or a baby who is under- or over-aroused (who is unresponsive), makes it more likely that his mother will subsequently become depressed.[8]

## ASSESSMENT

Postnatal depression is often under-detected and under-treated. The symptoms can easily be overlooked and attributed to tiredness, sleepless nights and the demands of coping with a baby. In addition, many mothers are reluctant to admit they are feeling down, or not really coping at this stage in their life when they are supposed to be happy and enjoying their new baby. Answers to questions may be influenced by a strong desire to appear a capable mother. Therefore, it is especially important to be sympathetic and non-judgemental when asking how she is feeling.

Firstly, look for the following symptoms of major depression.

➤ **Cognitive:** A negative view of one's self, the world and the future; poor concentration; sluggish thinking.
➤ **Affective:** Low mood; irritability; sometimes anxiety or agitation.
➤ **Behavioural:** Loss of interest in previously enjoyed interests and activities; social withdrawal; psychomotor retardation.
➤ **Biological:** Poor appetite; loss of weight; poor sleep; constipation; loss of libido.

Secondly, look for the following additional features.

➤ **Guilt:** A mother may be particularly guilty about feeling in despair at a time when she is supposed to be pleased with her new baby. She may conclude that she is a bad wife and mother.
➤ Obsessional thoughts.
➤ Fears of harming the baby.

### Differential diagnosis

Postnatal depression must be distinguished from the very common '*baby blues*', occurring towards the end of the first week; and *puerperal psychosis*, which requires urgent psychiatric referral and treatment because of risks to the baby. One way of thinking about postnatal depression is to see it as intermediate in severity between these two and distinct from both (*see* Table 14.1).

**TABLE 14.1** Causes of post-partum mood changes

| Disorder | Prevalence | Onset |
| --- | --- | --- |
| Baby blues | 30–50% | 3–7 days |
| Postnatal depression | At least 1 in 10 | 0–12 months |
| Puerperal Psychosis | About 1 per 1,000 | 1–4 weeks |

## Detection

Early detection is important. This cannot be done until the end of the first week or two, by which time the baby blues will have passed. Women may recognise there is something wrong, but few may think they have postnatal depression, and even fewer report how they feel to health professionals (unless asked).[9] Screening using the Edinburgh Postnatal Depression Scale has been shown to be an easy and reliable way of detecting postnatal depression.[10] It is a 10-item, self-report questionnaire with high specificity and sensitivity. It has been used and validated in clinical practice in primary care. Several studies have shown how easy it is for health visitors and general practitioners to use.[11] Each question is scored 0–3, according to increased severity of the symptom. Questions 1, 2 and 4 are scored 0-1-2-3, while questions 3, 5, 6, 7, 8, 9 and 10 are reverse scored 3-2-1-0. A score of 12 or above is an indicator of the need for further assessment. Some mothers may find the questions intrusive, and would prefer to talk about how they feel.[12] Whether or not this questionnaire is used, clinical assessment remains important.[13]

It has been suggested that two of these questions may be enough to screen for possible depression:[14]

➤ during the past month have you often been bothered by feeling down, depressed or hopeless?
➤ during the past month have you often been bothered by having little interest or pleasure in doing things?

If the answer to either of these questions is positive, a third question can be added:[15]
➤ is this something you feel you need or want help with?

However, this abbreviated format has not been adequately evaluated – in contrast to the full Edinburgh Postnatal Depression Scale, which has been extensively evaluated. The present authors therefore recommend continuing to use the full scale.

## MANAGEMENT[16]

### Primary prevention

Antenatal classes and the fostering of social support may help prevent postnatal depression, and should be widely available. A routine visit by the health visitor in the last trimester may help to encourage prospective mothers to attend antenatal and postnatal classes and form a relationship that may be invaluable later. A systematic review of psychosocial and psychological interventions for *preventing* postnatal depression found no evidence that any were effective.[17] Similarly, antidepressants are not recommended for the prophylaxis of postnatal depression, given the lack of clear evidence.[18]

### Secondary prevention of the effects on the child

Early detection of postnatal depression is essential. Despite increasing awareness of the extent and importance of postnatal depression, many cases are undetected or inadequately treated. Health visitors, general practitioners, paediatricians and

**TABLE 14.2** The Edinburgh Postnatal Depression Scale

| | |
|---|---|
| Name: ..........................  ...............................<br>Date filled in:......../ ......../ .........<br>Baby's age:.......... *weeks / months / years* | Cox JL, Holden JM, Sagovsky R. Detection of postnatal depression: development of the ten-item Edinburgh postnatal depression scale. *British Journal of Psychiatry.* 1987; **150**: 782–6. [To protect copyright, this must be quoted on all reproduced copies.] |

As you have recently had a baby, we would like to know how you are feeling. Please underline the answer that comes closest to how you have felt **in the past seven days** – not just how you feel today. Here is an example, already completed:

| | |
|---|---|
| I have felt happy:<br> Yes, all the time<br> Yes, most of the time<br> No, not very often<br> No, not at all | This would mean 'I have felt happy for most of the time' during the past week. Please complete the other questions in the same way. |

**In the past seven days:**

1 I have been able to laugh and see the funny side of things:
- as much as I always could
- not quite so much now
- definitely not so much now
- not at all.

2 I have looked forward with enjoyment to things:
- as much as I ever did
- rather less than I used to
- definitely less than I used to
- hardly at all.

3 I have blamed myself unnecessarily when things went wrong.
- Yes, most of the time.
- Yes, some of the time.
- Not very often.
- No, never.

4 I have been anxious or worried for no good reason.
- No, not at all.
- Hardly ever.
- Yes, sometimes.
- Yes, very often.

5 I have felt scared or panicky for no very good reason.
- Yes, quite a lot.
- Yes, sometimes.
- No, not much.
- No, not at all.

6 Things have been getting on top of me.
- Yes, most of the time I haven't been able to cope at all.
- Yes, sometimes I haven't been coping as well as usual.
- No, most of the time I have coped quite well.
- No, I have been coping as well as ever.

7 I have been so unhappy that I have been having difficulty sleeping.
- Yes, most of the time.
- Yes, sometimes.
- Not very often.
- No, not at all.

8 I have felt sad or miserable.
- Yes, most of the time
- Yes, quite often
- Not very often
- No, not at all.

9 I have been so unhappy that I have been crying.
- Yes, most of the time.
- Yes, quite often.
- Only occasionally.
- No, never.

10 The thought of harming myself has occurred to me.
- Yes, quite often.
- Sometimes.
- Hardly ever.
- Never.

others who come into contact should not feel embarrassed to ask women how they are feeling and coping, particularly if they are tearful. Routine screening using the Edinburgh Postnatal Depression Scale (or the above two to three questions)[19] should be carried out by the health visitor either during a routine home visit or when the baby has his development assessments. Asking about suicidal ideation and guilt may arouse strong feelings, but these questions are an essential part of the assessment, and women may feel a great sense of relief to share their concerns.

**BOX 14.1** Case Example

Louise is 25 years old when she comes to see her general practitioner three weeks after the birth of her first baby, Gemma, by ventouse (vacuum) delivery at 38 weeks gestation. She has been advised by the hospital to get a repeat blood test to check whether she needs to remain on iron tablets.

When the general practitioner asks Louise how she is getting along generally, Louise admits to feeling very tired and lacking in energy. She is not sleeping much; Gemma feeds from the breast on demand frequently throughout the night. Louise feels close to tears all the time, sometimes panicky and at times unable to cope, particularly when alone at night. Her husband is a shift-worker who sometimes works late in the evening and sometimes all night. She is getting only three-to-four hours sleep each night. During the day, she feels exhausted physically and mentally; she has noticed being very forgetful and unable to concentrate; and her appetite has not picked up since the exhaustion of her long labour. She admits to feeling frustrated at times with Gemma, but says she has managed to refrain from shouting at her, and has not even considered smacking her. On examination, the doctor thinks Louise looks clinically anaemic, so arranges for a full blood count and a measure of iron stores (ferritin). She asks Louise to come back a week later.

Later the same day, the general practitioner meets with the practice health visitor to discuss their joint concerns about Louise. Although the Edinburgh Postnatal Depression score is only 11, the general practitioner thinks she is quite depressed – and completely exhausted. The health visitor agrees that Louise seems depressed, but thinks she is taking good care of Gemma, who does not appear to be at any risk. The doctor reads from the old notes to the health visitor that Louise had a depressive episode two years ago, which responded well to antidepressants. They agree to monitor the situation closely, and the general practitioner agrees to discuss antidepressants at the next appointment.

The following week, Louise reports still being low and panicky at times. Her haemoglobin is slightly below the normal range at 10.3 g/dL, so the general practitioner prescribes her some iron tablets. Gemma is still feeding several times each night, so Louise has not been able to catch up on sleep. She is also worried that Gemma has not yet regained her birth weight. Louise remains very keen on breastfeeding; the general practitioner discusses the advantages and disadvantages of this. She also mentions the idea that antidepressants might help Louise as much as they have in the past, but Louise is worried about poisoning Gemma, and will not hear of it. They discuss how Louise could get some more sleep, and agree that she will have Gemma in bed with her so that Gemma can continue to feed on demand without waking Louise.

The general practitioner continues to see Louise weekly to monitor her depressive symptoms, and the health visitor also visits during the opposite half of the week. She discusses with Louise how she can involve her husband more with Gemma: he seems a bit scared of Gemma, and has hardly yet picked her up! Louise agrees to discuss this with him, and ask him to do practical tasks with Gemma, and play with her, in the gaps between his sleeps and his work shifts.

It turns out that Louise's husband is very willing to help, but was lacking in confidence. He missed most of the antenatal classes, because of his work patterns, but agrees to come to the daily mother-and-baby drop-in club when he can (about twice a week). He is very sympathetic to Louise's exhaustion (he knows what it is like) and works out a way of letting Louise have a nap during the day in-between feeds.

Louise continues on iron tablets, which make her constipated but gradually seem to build up her reserves of energy. She remains rather forgetful, with an erratic appetite, but is no longer panicky and only occasionally feels close to tears. She has worked out how to get some sleep when she has any opportunity. Gemma starts to put on weight. The general practitioner decides antidepressants are no longer necessary, so lengthens the gaps between Louise's appointments.

## Psychological interventions

A systematic review of psychological and psychosocial interventions concluded that peer support and non-directive counselling, cognitive behavioural therapy, psychodynamic psychotherapy, and interpersonal therapy are all effective in postnatal depression.[20]

Health visitors can learn a variety of brief psychological interventions targeted directly at the depressive mood, for instance based on the principles of cognitive behavioural therapy and person-centred active listening.[21,22,23] Interventions based on either of these treatment models can be cost-effective as part of a package of care.[24] Components of a health visitor intervention may include:

➤ an initial session lasting one hour in which the health visitor allows the mother to describe her current circumstances and emotional state
➤ subsequent fortnightly sessions lasting 30 minutes each (making a total of six sessions in three months)
➤ activity scheduling (the mother could for instance take the baby to the park, to mother-and-baby groups, or to show off to her friends)
➤ problem-solving practical difficulties about managing the child
➤ problem-solving relationship difficulties with the child, partner or extended family
➤ discussion of depressive thoughts and how to deal with them.

### The use of antidepressants[25]

Trials of antidepressants in pregnant or breastfeeding mothers are scarce: such mothers tend not to want to take medication. One trial found fluoxetine to be effective in comparison to placebo, whether combined with cognitive behavioural therapy or not.[26] Any treatment of benefit in non-postnatal depression should also be effective in postnatal depression.[27] The manufacturers of fluoxetine list lactation as a contraindication. There is also theoretical concern about the long half-life of fluoxetine causing accumulation in the baby. It seems that all antidepressants are present in breast milk, although sertraline has been found not to affect serotonin metabolism in the infant and is viewed as a good first choice for treatment-naive women:[28,29] sertraline and paroxetine are excreted in breast milk far less than fluoxetine and citalopram.[30] Lactating mothers are usually, quite appropriately, reluctant to give up breastfeeding. In practice, it is probably wisest to offer mothers the choice of a psychological intervention or antidepressants.[31] If antidepressants are chosen, then a selective serotonin reuptake inhibitor should probably be used first, such as sertraline or paroxetine, and the baby should be monitored regularly for sedation, irritability and any changes in the pattern of sleep, feeding or growth.

**BOX 14.2** Case Example

Helen, aged 35 years, is in regular contact with her health visitor following the birth of her first baby, Daniel. She wants to breastfeed, but is finding this problematic. The health visitor becomes concerned about Helen's mood as the weeks pass by: Helen increasingly presents in the baby clinic as tearful, and describes herself as feeling exhausted and getting little sleep. It seems that Helen and her partner have little family or social support – they have recently moved into the area. Helen also admits to the health visitor that she has had periods of despondency in the past, which she thinks may have been due to her setting rather high standards for herself.

The health visitor decides to meet Helen at home to discuss options for local support that may help Helen feel less isolated (and to further her assessment). Helen is then able to reveal how difficult it is to admit that she is not coping and how guilty she feels about not enjoying Daniel's company. She is very concerned about the impact this may have in the long-term as she is painfully aware that she is frequently irritable with Daniel and not always able to comfort him adequately. Helen also worries silently how her partner may perceive this. She states repeatedly that she should be able to cope. Helen describes occasional fleeting thoughts about taking an overdose. The health visitor is concerned that Helen is showing signs of depression, but is reassured that Daniel seems very well cared-for – in contrast to Helen's vitriolic self-criticism.

The health visitor asks Helen to complete the Edinburgh Postnatal Depression Scale. This gives a score of 18, indicating the need for further assessment. Helen sees her general practitioner the next day: he encourages her to continue attending the under-ones group at the health centre, and also discusses with her the option of antidepressants. The health visitor continues to meet with Helen at the family home, and explores with Helen how she could allow her partner to help her more, particularly during the night, so that she can reverse her sleep-deprivation. Helen reluctantly agrees to put Daniel onto one formula feed per night, to enable her partner to give at least one night feed.

Although Helen initially resists the idea of antidepressants, because of her desire to make a success of breastfeeding, the general practitioner encourages her at her next appointment to give them a try, since her mood has further deteriorated. He reassures her that sertraline is unlikely to be much present in breast milk, and the small quantities there may be are unlikely to do much to Daniel. Helen reluctantly agrees to start a low dose of sertraline and build it up gradually.

Over the next few months, Helen's mood gradually improves. She describes herself as having more energy. She is now meeting regularly with another mother from the under-ones group, which has helped her realise she is not the only mother struggling with a new baby.

The general practitioner continues to monitor Helen's mood and medication until Daniel is a year old, by which time Helen seems a lot more positive about everything, and has developed a more active social life, much of which includes her partner.

## The risk to the child

Part of the management of a mother with postnatal depression involves thinking about the risk to the child. At the very least, the child will experience the mother as less available and responsive – which affects the child's emotional and cognitive development.[32] More extreme risks to the child may develop, for instance if the mother becomes too depressed to be able to care effectively for the child, or if she develops an intention to harm the child. Mothers will usually admit to this intention if asked. In this situation, advice should be sought urgently from the local adult mental health team and social services' duty desk for children.

## REFERRAL

Indications for referral of a mother with postnatal depression to an adult mental health team include:
➤ current psychotic features
➤ a past history of puerperal psychosis, bipolar disorder or schizophrenia
➤ clearly planned suicidal intent
➤ well-formed intentions to harm the baby
➤ severe or worsening depression
➤ poor response to treatment.

## APPENDIX: A PERSONAL ACCOUNT OF POSTNATAL DEPRESSION[33]

*I was diagnosed as having postnatal depression when my son Louis was nine months old. My Doctor and health visitor had been 'watching me' since his birth. My daughter Connie was nine years old at this time. I think, hindsight being 20/20 vision, that I had postnatal depression when **she** was born: however, I blamed most of my*

**BOX 14.3** Practice Points about postnatal depression

Although common, it is often not recognised by mothers or professionals.

Sufferers may have a need to conceal their symptoms.

Important risk factors include a past psychiatric history and poor social support.

It is generally under-treated.

It can have significant long-term effects on both mother and child.

It therefore needs to be treated promptly.

A range of psychological therapies is effective in treating postnatal depression.

Most mothers are likely to prefer psychological treatments.

Antidepressants may be more readily available in some areas.

Health visitors and general practitioners have an important role in assessment and treatment.

Health visitors can give an effective brief psychological treatment.

General practitioners can prescribe antidepressants that are effective and probably safe.

Most cases can be managed in primary care and do not require referral.

*symptoms on an already failing first marriage. Fortunately, I am now in a very strong and happy marriage to my second husband, Pete.*

*I don't know whether there was one single reason for my depression, but I see it as a culmination of many factors, each of which on its own I would probably have been able to cope with. I had a happy and healthy pregnancy. Louis was 14 days overdue. He was induced, but went into foetal distress, and I was eventually given an emergency caesarean section, which I was obviously not prepared for. Louis was a very colicky baby and cried a lot. He also had eczema, caused by a milk allergy, which took approximately four months to be diagnosed.*

*At five months old, he became very ill and we had the doctor out to him every day for a week. He was not improving, and eventually he was taken into hospital. The next morning, the consultant saw Louis and told me he suspected meningitis. Louis had to have a lumbar puncture, and Pete had to hold him down while it was done. In fact Louis did have viral meningitis, and was in hospital for a week. I stayed with him the whole time. He left hospital with gastroenteritis and we watched his weight plummet over the following two weeks.*

*It was when Louis recovered that my health began to deteriorate.*

*I felt I was not the sort of person that this kind of thing happened to. I am usually a strong person – the kind others turn to in times of crisis. Like most people, I had a fear of mental illness, of not being in control of my own mind.*

*I simply was not coping with life. An example of this was when our kitchen ceiling was resurfaced. The man ripped our floor covering. Normally, I would have not paid him for the work, or would have negotiated some form of compensation. Due to the illness, I locked the children and myself in the living room, and refused to talk to him.*

*Pete was so taken aback by this behaviour that he simply paid the workman to get him out of the way so he could calm me.*

*I became very withdrawn: I would not leave the house unless I really had to. I couldn't answer the telephone; I would let the answering machine take the call, and maybe then pick the call up or get Pete to phone the person back later. Connie was in on this system. When she was in, she would answer the telephone and tell the caller that I was unavailable.*

*Connie and I have always had a very close relationship. We spent five years on our own as a 'two family'. She has always been protective of me even when I really didn't need protecting. She will not have a bad word said against me and frequently tells me I am the best or most cool mum.*

*During the depths of my depression, Connie and I almost swapped roles. She became very protective of me and would act as a cushion from the outside world. She became the parent and I the child. She grew up a lot in the first two years of Louis' life. Some of this must be due to the fact that she was no longer the one and only but now a big sister, and some must be due to her age: she was at an age when you go from being a little girl to a young lady. However, I do know that some of the explanation must be living with me during my depression.*

*We are a family that communicates well. We discuss most things openly and Connie was a party to many discussions on how I was feeling and what others could do to help me. Her help was invaluable.*

*I could not go shopping alone, and still have problems in this area. I suffered from major panic attacks when out shopping and I relied on my family to help me. Both Pete and Connie coached me through the panic attacks, standing with me helping me to control my breathing. I still get panic attacks, mostly associated with shopping in town, but I am able to deal with them myself as they are far less severe than those I initially experienced.*

*I really hit an all-time low when my doctor told me I was clinically depressed. Until this point I was kidding myself that I was not that bad, even though I was suffering from some very severe symptoms. The main reason that I considered my depression not to be severe was because I felt no animosity towards Louis; I loved him from the moment he was laid in my arms. I thought that all mothers with postnatal depression rejected their babies. I learnt from the other mothers that I contacted through the locally run postnatal depression support group that this was far from true.*

*Looking at us now I feel as a family we have benefited from the depression. We are strong and definitely more understanding of illness in others.*

*As for the effect on Louis, I think each thing that happens to a child goes towards developing their character. Louis is a happy, social child who interacts well with both adults and his peers. As I had returned to full-time working prior to my sick leave, he benefited from nine months of my company, and his company made me strong at times when I might have gone to pieces on my own. After my sick leave I returned to work on a part time basis, and this continues, so that Louis and I spend time together still. He is a mummy's boy, but no more than other children whose mothers have not been through depression.*

## RESOURCES

### Organisations that can help parents

- **National Childbirth Trust:** www.nct.org.uk
- **Association for Post-Natal Illness:** www.apni.org
- **Depression Alliance:** This is a charity for people with depression. www.depressionalliance. org
- **Gingerbread:** This is a national network of local groups providing single parents with support, friendship and social activities. www.gingerbread.org.uk
- **The Family Welfare Association:** In some areas of the UK, this helps families with children under five, and describes itself as 'a service for parents with mental health problems'. www. fwa.org.uk
- **Netmums**: This is a community support website for parents. www.netmums.com
- **SureStart**: This government programme to support young children and their parents runs a network of children's centres offering support, child health advice, and childcare. www. surestart.gov.uk
- **Homestart UK**: This is a charity for families with children under five. www.home-start. org.uk
- **Twins and Multiple Births Association (TAMBA)**: This organisation supports families with twins, triplets or more through local Twins Clubs and specialist support groups. www.tamba. org.uk

### Reading for parents

- BBC online. *Postnatal Depression.* Available at: www.bbc.co.uk/parenting/having_a_baby/birth_pnd.shtml (accessed 26 March 2011).
- Cloutte P, Darton K. *Understanding Postnatal Depression.* London: MIND; 2008. Available at: www.mind.org.uk/help/diagnoses_and_conditions/post-natal_depression (accessed 26 March 2011).
- Gilbert P. *Overcoming Depression: a guide to recovery with a complete self-help programme.* London: Robinson; 2009.
- Hanzak EA. *Eyes Without Sparkle: a journey through postnatal illness.* Oxford: Radcliffe, 2005.
- Royal College of Psychiatrists. *Postnatal mental health: A combination of information resources.* London: Royal College of Psychiatrists; 2007. Available at: www.rcpsych.ac.uk/mentalhealthinfoforall/problems/postnatalmentalhealth.aspx (accessed 26 March 2011).
- Welford H. *Feelings after Birth: the NCT book of postnatal depression.* London: NCT Publishers; 2002.
- Wheatley SL. *Coping with Postnatal Depression (Overcoming Common Problems).* London: Sheldon Press; 2005.

### BOOK FOR PROFESSIONALS

- Milgrom J, Martin PR, Negri LM. *Treating Postnatal Depression: a psychological approach for healthcare practitioners.* Chichester and Oxford: Wiley-Blackwell; 1999.

### REFERENCES

1 Cooper PJ, Murray L. Prediction, detection and treatment of postnatal depression. *Arch Dis Child.* 1997; **77**(2): 97–9.

2 Murray L, Cooper PJ. Effects of postnatal depression on infant development. *Arch Dis Child.* 1997; **77**(2): 99–101.

3 Sharp D, Hay DF, Pawlby S, *et al.* The impact of postnatal depression on boys' intellectual development. *J Child Psychol Psychiatry.* 1995; **36**(8): 1315–36.

4 Luoma I, Tamminen T, Kaukonen P, *et al.* Longitudinal study of maternal depressive symptoms and child well-being. *J Am Acad of Child Adolesc Psychiatry.* 2001; **40**(12): 1367–74.

5 Avan B, Richter L, Ramchandani P, *et al.* Maternal postnatal depression and children's growth and behaviour during the early years of life: exploring the interaction between physical and mental health. *Arch Dis Child.* 2010; **95**(9): 690–5.

6 Warner R, Appleby L, Whitton A, *et al.* Demographic and obstetric risk factors for postnatal psychiatric morbidity. *Br J Psychiatry.* 1996; **168**(5): 607–11.

7 Musters C, McDonald E, Jones I. Management of postnatal depression. *BMJ.* 2008; **337**: a736.

8 Murray L, Stanley C, Hooper R, *et al.* The role of infant factors in postnatal depression and mother-infant interactions. *Dev Med Child Neurol.* 1996; **38**(2): 109–19.

9 Whitton A, Warner R, Appleby L. The pathway to care in post-natal depression: women's attitudes to post-natal depression and its treatment. *Br J Gen Pract.* 1996; **46**(408): 427–8.

10 Cox JL, Holden JM, Sagovsky R. Detection of postnatal depression: development of the ten-item Edinburgh Postnatal Depression Scale. *Br J Psychiatry.* 1987; **150**: 782–6.

11 Davies BR, Howells S, Jenkins M. Early detection and treatment of postnatal depression in primary care. *J Adv Nurs.* 2003; **44**(3): 248–55.

12 Shakespeare J, Blake F, Garcia J. A qualitative study of the acceptability of routine screening of postnatal women using the Edinburgh Postnatal Depression Scale. *Br J Gen Pract.* 2003; **53**(493): 614–19.

13 Pawlby S, Sharp D, Hay D, *et al.* Postnatal depression and child outcome at 11 years: the importance of accurate diagnosis. *J Affect Disord.* 2008; **107**(1–3): 241–5.

14 Whooley M, Avins A, Miranda J, *et al.* Case-finding instruments for depression: two questions are as good as many. *J Gen Intern Med.* 1997; **12**: 439–45.

15 National Institute for Health and Clinical Excellence. Antenatal and postnatal mental health: clinical management and service guidance [Clinical guideline 45]. London: NICE; 2007. Available at: http://guidance.nice.org.uk/CG45/NICEGuidance/pdf/English (accessed 26 March 2011).

16 Musters, op. cit.

17 Dennis CL, Creedy D. Psychosocial and psychological interventions for preventing postnatal depression. *Cochrane Database Syst Rev.* 2004 Oct 18; (4): CD001134.

18 Howard LM, Hoffbrand S, Henshaw C, *et al.* Antidepressant prevention of postnatal depression. *Cochrane Database Syst Rev.* 2005 Apr 18; (2): CD004363.

19 National Institute for Health and Clinical Excellence, op. cit.

20 Dennis CL, Hodnett E. Psychosocial and psychological interventions for treating postpartum depression. *Cochrane Database Syst Rev.* 2007; (4): CD006116.

21 Appleby L, Hirst E, Marshall S, *et al.* The treatment of postnatal depression by health visitors: impact of brief training on skills and clinical practice. *J Affect Disord.* 2003; **77**(3): 261–6.

22 Hawton K, Salkovskis PM, Kirk J, *et al. Cognitive Behaviour Therapy for Psychiatric Problems: a practical guide.* Oxford: Oxford University Press; 1989.

23 Egan G. *The Skilled Helper* [international edition]. California: Wadsworth; 2009.

24 Morrell CJ, Slade P, Warner R, *et al.* Clinical effectiveness of health visitor training in psychologically informed approaches for depression in postnatal women: pragmatic cluster randomised trial in primary care. *BMJ.* 2009; **338**: a3045.

25 Drug and Therapeutics Bulletin. The management of postnatal depression. *DTB.* 2000; **38**(5): 33–7.

26 Appleby L, Warner R, Whitton A, *et al.* A controlled study of fluoxetine and cognitive-behavioural counselling in the treatment of postnatal depression. *BMJ.* 1997; **314**: 932–6.

27 National Institute for Health and Clinical Excellence, op. cit.

28 Epperson CN, Anderson GM, McDougle CJ. Sertraline and breast feeding. *N Engl J Med.* 1997; **336**(16): 1189–90.

29 Whitby DH, Smith KM. The use of tricyclic antidepressants and selective serotonin reuptake inhibitors in women who are breast feeding. *Pharmacotherapy.* 2005: **25**(3): 411–25.

30 Weissman AM, Levy BT, Hartz AJ, *et al.* Pooled analysis of antidepressant levels in lactating mothers, breast milk, and nursing infants. *Am J Psychiatry.* 2004; **161**(6): 1066–78.

31 Appleby, op. cit.

32 Murray, 1997, op. cit.

33 We are indebted to Karen King of Worthing, West Sussex, for permission to publish this account of her own experience of postnatal depression.

# CHAPTER 15

# Crying and colic

## INTRODUCTION

Crying is one of the most powerful ways in which an infant can attract adult attention. Crying is part of the normal developmental process and serves several functions:

➤ a response to physiological discomforts such as hunger, pain or feeling uncomfortable

➤ an expression of emotional distress, such as fear or anxiety

➤ a communication with the caregiver, indicating a need to be met by them.

However functional it may be, crying – particularly inconsolable crying lasting for many hours – can be a cause of great distress to parents. As a result of this, crying is a frequent source of concern and parents often seek advice about it.

Excessive crying is a common problem: estimates of prevalence rates vary from 14–35% of babies.[1,2]

## CAUSES OF CRYING

### Three-month colic, persistent evening crying or evening fretting

It is difficult to arrive at a clear definition of *three-month colic*, and its aetiology is not fully understood. An alternative term is *persistent evening crying*. In general, colic is accepted to be a pattern of inconsolable crying occurring on a daily basis, often in the afternoon or evening, between about three and 14 weeks. Babies with colic tend to scream intensely for long periods, draw their legs up and look pale. Colic is a self-limiting condition occurring in babies who are thriving and otherwise well.

More commonly and less severely, the baby grizzles during the evening but is pacified relatively easily by being carried around or taken for a car ride. This is often called *evening fretting* and probably reflects the baby's inability to soothe himself and therefore his reliance on caregivers to comfort him.

There are a number of theories about the causes of colic, none of which have been proven. One of the most popular, at least amongst lay people, is that colic may be due to immaturity of the gut causing intestinal spasm. This theory is supported by the fact that antispasmodic drug therapy is the only medication that has been shown to have a therapeutic effect, and that premature babies who develop colic tend to do so within two weeks of the due date, regardless of gestation.

**BOX 15.1** Case Example

Sunita brings her four-month-old baby daughter, Padma, to clinic to see the health visitor. Sunita is very tearful and reports that Padma is continuously crying, particularly in the early evenings, making Sunita exhausted and very cross with Padma. The health visitor arranges to see Sunita at home to discuss the situation in more detail the next day.

Sunita is living in a first-floor flat. Her husband works shifts and does not come home until 9 pm most nights. Her mother lives nearby and is supportive. Padma was initially a very good baby and has started crying in the evenings only recently.

The health visitor reviews with Sunita the evening routine. She reassures Sunita that there seems to be nothing physically wrong with Padma and that she is putting on weight and developing normally.

Sunita has been settling Padma down in her crib in the sitting room with the television on after her evening feed. The health visitor suggests they start to establish a quieter routine with Padma being settled in her crib after a feed in her parents' bedroom. The health visitor also suggests that Sunita should remove one of the blankets from the crib, as she suspects Padma may be too hot.

The health visitor encourages Sunita to leave Padma in the crib – even if she is crying – for up to 20 minutes to see if she settles. Sunita agrees with the health visitor that she would find it helpful to have her mother around until her husband comes home. The health visitor suggests that, if Sunita feels cross, she should take some time out away from the baby and leave her to cry.

They review the situation after a few days. Sunita's mother reports that Padma is vomiting some of her feed and seems uncomfortable after her feed. The health visitor discusses this with the general practitioner and they then recommended a week's trial of a soya feed.

There seems to be an improvement in the crying after this change, although Padma still tends to be more irritable in the early evenings. Sunita is however able to tolerate this and establishes a quiet, calm evening routine that enables her to feel more in control of the situation and less likely to get so upset herself.

## Hunger

One of the commonest reasons for frequent or near continual crying in a young baby is hunger. Weighing and plotting on a growth chart is a simple exercise, to assess whether the baby is in fact being adequately nourished. On the other hand, mothers who breastfeed sometimes give up unnecessarily because they fear their baby's crying is a sign of hunger when it is not.

## Diet

The pattern of crying is different in formula-fed to breast-fed babies.[3] Formula–fed babies cry more at two weeks of age, while breastfed babies cry more and sleep less at six weeks of age. Cow's milk protein is often implicated in colic, but soya-based milks are not necessarily better: a hypoallergenic formula may be necessary.[4] Concerns have been expressed – with much anecdotal evidence – about substances transmitted in breast milk causing crying in the infant (for instance, cow's milk, caffeine, spices, brassicas, chocolate and beans).

### Wind

Crying following a feed is often thought to be due to wind. According to this lay theory, it can be terminated by burping manoeuvres. A related theory is that wind can be caused by bottle-feeding from a teat with too large a hole, but clinical practice suggests that changing teat size does not lead to a dramatic improvement.

### Illness

Many parents feel that their inconsolable crying baby must be in pain and therefore ill. Colic will probably be implicated in the majority of these cases, and the child will be physically well. A common cause of colic is cow's milk allergy. However, it is obviously important not to miss the less common causes of excessive crying, such as pain from acute infections (ear, nose and throat, or urinary tract) or from a strangulated inguinal (groin) hernia. Crying after a feed may be due to pain from gastro-oesophageal reflux, and this may be associated with unusual posturing of the baby's head and neck. There will usually (but not always) be a history of vomiting. If suspected, this possibility should be investigated by a paediatrician. A rare but extremely important condition is infantile seizures, where the baby flexes the whole trunk in a so-called 'salaam' spasm and utters a brief cry. A child with possible infantile spasms should probably be referred as an emergency.

**BOX 15.2** Practice Points for the management of excessive crying in infants

The majority of infant crying is self-limiting with no long-term sequelae.

Allow parents space to express their concerns and listen to them carefully.

Do not underestimate the stress that an inconsolably crying child can cause in a family.

A diary may be very helpful to complete the assessment and assess the impact of any interventions.

As there is no single proven solution to the problem, be flexible and offer parents a range of management options.

Brainstorm a list of common-sense solutions, such as:
- offering a feed to the baby when she cries
- non-nutritive sucking
- holding
- rocking
- soothing sounds
- taking the baby for a drive in the car.

Try reducing stimulation, particularly for tense babies, and increasing stimulation for active babies.

Try for one week replacing cow's milk formula with hypoallergenic formula.

Ensure appropriate support for parents is available, preferably from the extended family.

Parents may need professional support in addition.

Referral to a paediatrician may be necessary for social and/or medical reasons.

Referral to social care may be necessary if parents are so desperate and so unsupported that abuse seems a risk.

### Birth complications and prematurity

The reputed Chinese aphorism 'difficult birth, difficult child' has a grain of truth. Babies who have had complicated and traumatic deliveries have been shown to be more irritable and cry more,[5] as have premature and low birth weight babies.[6] The nature of their cries is also reported to be high pitched and irritating and so more distressing to parents.

### Temperament

Temperamental changes are associated with the amount and style of an infant's crying. Two temperamental groups that may cause particular problems are those babies that appear tense and dislike handling and stimulation, and active babies who seem to demand much attention and stimulation.

### Parental anxiety or stress

It has been suggested that anxiety and tension in a parent may contribute to her baby's crying. First babies cry more than second, but this may simply be a reflection of the fact that first-time parents are often more aware of crying and less skilled at preventing it. It is also very difficult to separate cause from effect, as parents whose baby cries inconsolably will tend to be tenser than parents with a contented infant – not least because of sleep deprivation due to night-time crying.

### ASSESSMENT

By the time parents of crying babies approach a professional, they may have already received a vast amount of conflicting advice from friends and relatives, and be feeling bewildered and inadequate. It is extremely important to allow them space to discuss their anxieties and to avoid appearing judgmental if you are to maintain a therapeutic relationship.

The aim of assessment is to try to help the parents to see the problem in a systematic way, so they can approach solutions in a logical fashion.

### An approach to assessment

➤ *Consider medical problems.*

Inquire about any signs of physical illness, including fever, and recommend an assessment with the general practitioner if there are any signs of the baby being unwell.

➤ *Obtain a detailed description of the crying.*
Ask about the age at which crying started.
Have there been any periods of improvement or deterioration?
Is there a pattern to the crying – best and worst times of day, intensity and duration?
What methods have the parents used to try to control the crying?
Which have been successful?
➤ *Feeding.*
Breast or bottle or both? Quality of sucking.
Length, volume and frequency of feeds.
Relation of crying to feeding.
➤ *Sleeping.*
Pattern of sleeping during day and night.
Relation to feeding.
➤ *Psychosocial factors.*
What effect does the child's crying have on the parents?
What do they fear may be wrong?
How tense and irritable have they felt; do they ever fear they may get frustrated and harm the baby?
Is the mother becoming depressed?
What sort of support is there for the mother, from father, extended family or neighbours?

### A CRYING DIARY

It may be difficult for parents to recall accurately the pattern of crying. It may seem to a stressed mother that her baby screams constantly, when in fact there are a number of screaming episodes occurring unpredictably throughout the day. It is often very helpful to ask parents to fill in a diary for a few days, in which they record accurate details of crying episodes (time, duration, intensity, exacerbating or relieving factors and parents' responses), as well as sleeping and feeding patterns (*see* Table 15.1). This technique also has the advantage of saving a considerable amount of time in the consultation, if time constraints are a factor. It also helps identify strategies that help to reduce the crying (a tired parent will often say that nothing works) and can be used to monitor the effects of different techniques.

### MANAGEMENT

The majority of problems with crying babies are self-limiting and have no serious long-term consequences (although they may cause severe stress and distress within the family in the short-term). In general, these babies lend themselves very well to management without referral, for instance by the health visitor or family support worker. If more than one professional becomes involved, professional discussions may be necessary to ensure that advice is coordinated rather than conflicting.

**TABLE 15.1** Example of a crying diary

| Day and date | Crying episode: beginning and ending times | How loud was it (on a scale of 0–5)? | Time of last sleep before crying | Time of last feed before crying | What did you do? | What made it better? | What made it worse? |
|---|---|---|---|---|---|---|---|
|  |  |  |  |  |  |  |  |
|  |  |  |  |  |  |  |  |
|  |  |  |  |  |  |  |  |
|  |  |  |  |  |  |  |  |
|  |  |  |  |  |  |  |  |
|  |  |  |  |  |  |  |  |
|  |  |  |  |  |  |  |  |

### Reassurance

Many parents of crying babies believe that the terrible wails must reflect a serious underlying medical problem. They will be helped by perceiving that their worries have been taken seriously, and that the baby has been adequately examined. If they bring the baby to a health professional such as the general practitioner or health visitor, examination is therefore important even if the professional feels sure from the history that there is no physical problem.

For some parents, reassurance that there is nothing physically wrong with the baby, and that the crying will resolve spontaneously with no long-term ill effects, will be enough to solve the problem. For others, further advice on management is needed (*see* below).

In some cases, such as when a baby cries persistently during the day, the label of a 'difficult temperament' may be more helpful than that of 'three-month colic'. This takes the blame away from the parents without inferring any organic cause. This label is particularly useful for babies who also have sleeping and feeding problems.

### Routines

Experience at a 'crying clinic' where diaries were used suggested that relevant factors in some cases included a lack of routine or a lack of understanding by the parents of the baby's needs.[7] Providing simple, clear advice on feeding (volume, timing and techniques) and sleeping patterns (settling routines and naps) seemed to help these parents.

In another treatment trial,[8] parents were advised to go through a checklist in response to the baby's crying:

Could he be hungry?
Does he want to suck (without being hungry)?
Does he want to be held?
Is he bored and wanting stimulation?
Does he want to go to sleep?

Parents were advised to try each response for five minutes in turn, and not to worry about overfeeding or spoiling the baby. This resulted in a 70% improvement in crying. Both these studies emphasised the value of diaries in assessment and providing feedback to parents and health professionals.

### Specific interventions

#### Rhythmic movement

Rocking has been used to still crying babies for centuries and is often effective. Rates of around 60 rocks per minute seem to be most soothing – interestingly this is the speed of comfortable rocking in a rocking chair. Carrying the baby while walking at a rate of one step per second, pushing in a pram or driving in a car may also be useful.

#### Soothing sound

Soft, rhythmic singing of lullabies is also a tried and tested method. It has been shown that continuous sound will decrease the arousal level of infants. Modern equivalents include tapes of womb music and white noise emitters or the sound of an electrical appliance such as a washing machine, hair dryer or vacuum cleaner.

### Non-nutritive sucking

Sucking is often an extremely effective way of comforting babies, even if they are not hungry, and many babies seem to need to suck for far longer than is necessary for feeding. Many mothers instinctively do this by offering the breast. However, non-nutritive sucking by encouraging the baby to suck his hand or a dummy is also a potent calming method. A number of mothers and health professionals are anxious that the baby may become addicted to the dummy or harmed by its use. The main concerns expressed are that sucking a dummy will cause prominence of the front teeth: this becomes a potential problem only if the dummy is used excessively in older children (of three years and above). The other concern is that using a dummy will delay a child's language or cognitive development; however, if the dummy is used only when the baby wants it, rather than to stop every cry – which may inhibit communication – there is no evidence of long-term harm.

### Position

Many babies seem to be happiest in a particular position. Some mothers find that constantly carrying the baby in a sling is very helpful. This may be due to a combination of movement, stimulation and proximity to the (warmth and smell of) mother. Colicky babies are often more comfortable in a position that exerts gentle pressure on the abdomen by lying the baby with his tummy over an arm, knee or pillow or carrying the baby with his trunk slightly flexed. Tense babies like to be held firmly and not over-handled. They often respond well to being tightly wrapped in a sheet – a version of swaddling – whereas active babies generally prefer to be upright.

### Stimulation level

In a similar vein, these tense babies respond badly to overstimulation, and it can be helpful to keep activities such as nappy changes, bathing and undressing to a minimum. Active babies appear to demand stimulation and like to be constantly on the move, so devices such as baby bouncers can help, as can frequent walks, books, pictures and mobiles (pretty objects on strings – not phones).

Those babies who are unable to regulate their own level of arousal will cry excessively because they are tired and unable to settle themselves to sleep. Helping parents to recognise this can be beneficial, often by using diaries, so that rather than picking the baby up at the first moan, they wait several minutes to allow the baby the opportunity to learn to settle himself. In general, lessening stimulation has been found effective.[9]

### Dietary interventions

Elimination of cow's milk protein in bottle-fed babies can improve colic. A week's trial of a hypoallergenic formula can be used as a diagnostic test.[10] Substitution with soya milk is not reliable. Breastfed babies may cry less if supplemented with probiotics.[11] Lactating mothers have also been advised to eliminate cow's milk protein from their diet for a week to see if this relieves the baby's symptoms. It has been suggested that herbal teas such as camomile, fennel and balm mint, if taken by the mother, may be calming for the baby.

## Medication

Many parents attempt to use medicines to soothe crying babies. The most commonly used is gripe water, although there is no good research-based evidence to show that it works. In the past, dicyclomine (Merbentyl – an antispasmodic) was the most effective medication for colic. It is no longer recommended for babies under six months because of concern about rare respiratory and neurological side effects. Infacol contains dimeticone, which is an antifoaming agent claimed to relieve flatulence, although its value is uncertain. If a crying baby is thought to be suffering from reflux, there may be some value in trying to thicken feeds or use antacid preparations. In general, there is no clear research-based evidence that any of the currently available medicines are effective in crying babies.

## Support

Any parent can be driven to desperation by an inconsolably crying baby, to the point of fearing she may harm the child. In some cases, these feelings may be linked to memories of a difficult pregnancy, a painful labour or even an abusive childhood. It is also relevant to ask the parent of a seemingly difficult baby about the symptoms of depression (*see* Chapter 14 on Postnatal Depression). In extreme situations, physical abuse may result, but this is usually in socially isolated families.

It is essential to ensure that parents have enough support from each other, their extended family and their friends. The health visitor may be able to help by introduction to a mother and baby group or a local postnatal group. Support from volunteers, some of whom may have been through similar difficulties, can be obtained through voluntary organisations such as Homestart, Cry-sis and the National Childbirth Trust, all of which have useful websites with lots of advice and management strategies (*see* below, under Resources).

Parents can be advised that, if they reach a point at which they feel unable to cope with the crying, the best thing to do is put the baby in the safety of his cot, shut the door, go to another part of the house and if possible get help or support, even if this is only over the telephone. However, many parents feel too guilty to leave the child alone in this way, but may take on board advice that they must look after themselves in order to cope with the baby's demands.

In some cases a break can be offered by a member of the extended family temporarily taking care of the baby in order to give the full time carer a good night's rest. Parents can feel very guilty about doing this and should be encouraged to use the support of their extended family and be helped to see this as a positive action.

## REFERRAL

Babies with a serious underlying medical problem should be under the care of a paediatrician, and occasionally a paediatric assessment may be helpful to diffuse anxiety.

Sometimes a short break is necessary for carers, and a paediatric ward may agree to admit the infant for observation, to break the vicious cycle of anxiety and exhaustion. This also has the advantage of: assessing for any physical illness, (usually) effectively reassuring parents that there is none, revealing patterns of family interaction, and allowing some further psychosocial assessment.

When there is thought to be a risk of physical abuse to the child then a referral to social services should be made. This is more likely to occur in families who are unused to asking for help and are isolated.

## RESOURCES

### Further reading

- Kitzinger S. *Understanding Your Crying Baby: why babies cry, how parents feel and what you can do about it.* London: Carroll & Brown Publishers Limited; 2005.
- Lester BM, Grace CO. *Why Is My Baby Crying? The parent's survival guide for coping with crying problems and colic.* London: HarperCollins Publishers; 2006.
- Mulholland S. *Coping with Crying and Colic: an easy-to-follow guide.* London: Vermilion; 2008.

### Support groups

- Cry-sis: www.cry-sis.org.uk
- Home Start: www.home-start.org.uk
- Sure Start: www.education.gov.uk/childrenandyoungpeople/earlylearningandchildcare/sure start
- Family Action: www.family-action.org.uk
- National Childbirth Trust: www.nct.org.uk/home
- NSPCC: helpline 0808 800 5000; www.nspcc.org.uk

## REFERENCES

1 Butler NR, Golding J. *From Birth to Five: a study of health and behaviour in Britain's five-year-olds.* London: Pergamon Press; 1986.
2 Thomas DB. Aetiological associations in infantile colic: an hypothesis. *Aust Paediatr J.* 1981; **17**: 292–5.
3 Lucas A, St James-Roberts I. Crying, fussing and colic behaviour in breast- and bottle-fed infants. *Early Hum Dev.* 1998; **53**(1): 9–18.
4 Lucassen PL, Assendelft WJ, Gubbels W, *et al.* Effectiveness of treatments for infantile colic: systematic review. *BMJ.* 1998; **316**(7144): 1563–9 [published erratum appears in: *BMJ.* 1998; **317**: 171].
5 Thomas, op. cit.
6 Butler, op. cit.
7 Pritchard. An infant crying clinic. *Health Visit.* 1986; **59**(12): 375–7.

8 Taubman B. Clinical trial of the treatment of colic by modification of parent-infant interaction. *Pediatrics.* 1984; **74**(6): 998–1003.

9 Lucassen, op. cit.

10 Ibid.

11 Savino F, Pelle E, Palumeri E, *et al.* Lactobacillus reuteri (American Type Culture Collection Strain 55730) versus simethicone in the treatment of infantile colic: a prospective randomized study. *Pediatrics.* 2007; **119**(1): e124–30.

# CHAPTER 16

# Feeding in babies and toddlers

## INTRODUCTION

Feeding problems in preschool children are extremely common. About 10% of young children will demonstrate some problem with food refusal at some stage during their childhood: possibly a third of five year olds have a mild to moderate eating problem.[1] The vast majority of these children are thriving and will outgrow their feeding problem with no long-term ill effects, but parents can nevertheless become disproportionally anxious. This is probably because the refusal of food feels like a challenge to the parents' abilities to nurture their child and fully meet his needs at a most basic level. The child's refusal to eat can feel from a parent's point of view to be rejecting – and perhaps hurtful – so can lead to significant family worries about mealtimes and the child's overall diet. A parent may also experience a food-refusing child (usually of three to five years) as controlling in such a way as to demonstrate – to the parent and anyone who is watching – how poorly she performs as a parent.

## ASSESSMENT

When a parent presents with a problem related to feeding, a proper assessment of the situation is essential.

### History

*History of the presenting complaint.* What exactly is worrying the parent? Is the child faddy, refusing food, not eating at the table or behaving unacceptably? Is there real concern that the child is not thriving?

*An account of a typical meal.* Do meals occur at a regular time with a reliable pattern? Which foods is the child being offered and how large are the portions? Does the family sit down and eat to provide an example, or are there multiple distractions such as people coming and going or confusing commands being given? What is the duration of the meal: is there a sense of rush? Are the parents coercive, tending to be punitive in their handling of the child and noting all that the child does wrong? How does the child behave? Can anyone feed the child successfully?

*Parental expectations and attitudes towards food.* Are there unrealistic expectations of the amount of food a small child requires? What conscious or unconscious views are held by parents? For instance: 'Babies should be fat'; 'Food equals love' or 'The plate must always be clean'. Is there criticism from grandparents? Are there parental memories of having battles over food as children?

*Dietary history.* When was the child weaned from breast milk/from bottled milk/onto solids? What are the child's favourite things to eat? Are there any foods he particularly dislikes? Does the child drink a lot of milk or sugary drinks? Does the child eat between meals? Parents often initially deny this, but close questioning may reveal considerable amounts of snacks and sweets being offered to make up for refused meals. Supplementary bottles of milk may be offered to the child in an effort to make sure he is getting enough nourishment. Do other family members slip the child sweets and food?

*Developmental history.* Both overall development delay and specific developmental problems such as speech delay may be associated with feeding problems. The association with speech delay is due to the frequent link to oral-motor dysfunction. Sensory problems, such as excessive sensitivity to smell and taste, even without a diagnosable developmental disorder, may also be associated with feeding difficulties (*see also* Chapter 32).

*Medical history.* Is there any suggestion of an organic cause for failure to thrive, such as chronic illness or malabsorption? Is the child taking any medication that could suppress appetite, such as methylphenidate for ADHD? A past history of choking or vomiting, particularly if associated with oesophageal reflux, may lead to continuing feeding difficulties even after the choking or vomiting has long stopped; this may be due to aversive conditioning in the child – feeding is linked to unpleasant experiences, such as the pain of acid coming up from the stomach – combined with the resulting parental anxiety.

*Family and social history.* Were there similar problems or any history of eating disorders in other family members? Have there been any recent traumatic events that could have triggered these problems, such as the arrival of a new sibling, maternal depression, departure of a partner or loss of a grandparent?

### Examination

The majority of children presenting with feeding disorders are physically normal and thriving, but a small percentage may have rare medical problems. It is important not to miss these few children who may be genuinely failing to thrive. It is also important to provide informed reassurance to the majority of parents whose child is growing normally. The child's weight and height should always be plotted on a centile chart with explanation to the parents, ideally with previous readings for comparison. A general medical examination should assess nutritional status and ensure that the palate is intact: this can be done initially by the general practitioner.

### A food diary

It is often very helpful to ask the carer to fill in a food diary for a few days. All food eaten is recorded (it is important to stress that as well as meals the diary should include snacks such as sweets, crisps and biscuits). It is also important to include food that is refused and information about mealtime behaviour. As well as providing useful information for the health professional, these diaries are often reassuring to the carer, who may see that the child is eating more than she had realised.

The diary also provides an opportunity to offer simple common sense advice about nutrition and behaviour, which may be all that is necessary.

## Observation

If it is possible to observe a meal in person or to watch a video of mealtimes recorded by the family, much useful information can be obtained. If a video is used it can also be played back to the parent to illustrate interactions. For instance, if the child refuses food and gets a strong reaction from the parent, the child is likely to continue to do this.

## MANAGEMENT

### Weaning problems

Babies are commonly weaned from a milk-only diet to one including solids at about six months of age. Introducing solids at this stage seems to be important for the full development of chewing skills, and if the introduction of solids is delayed until much later, lumpy food may be rejected or vomited. There is also some evidence to suggest that presenting a range of foods and tastes at six months, and persisting in re-offering a refused food at subsequent meals is important in preventing the development of faddiness.[2]

### *Reluctance to give up breast or bottle*

The age at which parents want a baby to give up the breast or bottle varies greatly. One of the most important things to ensure is that the mother is clear in her motivation, rather than ambivalent. Various conflicting factors may affect the mother's decision, such as: cultural influences, pressures from family or friends, or the importance for the child (or mother) of comfort-sucking.

In general, a gradual but firm approach works best, with a limit established on the number of feeds rather than continual demand feeding. It can help to discuss how to do this and offer suggestions for alternative comforting such as giving drinks in a teacher-beaker, allowing finger-sucking or providing a teddy or blanket. Once a routine has been established, the mother can gradually drop feeds by reducing the number per day and increasing other sources of fluid. It is important to stress that once a feed has been dropped it should not be re-introduced in a moment of weakness.

### *Reluctance to chew lumps*

This often develops if solids have been introduced too late, so primary health care teams can offer important preventive advice to new parents about the timing of weaning. This problem can also sometimes be related to an episode when a child has choked or vomited on a lump and developed a fear of a repeat episode (aversive conditioning). If a child will take only puréed food then a gradual introduction of texture is best, adding substances such as flour, rice or potato until the food reaches the texture of mashed potato. Finger foods can also be introduced: licking spreads or jam off bread or biscuits can be a first step towards solids. Similarly,

**TABLE 16.1** Example of a food diary

| Day | Food eaten at breakfast | What happened at breakfast? | Snacks and drinks | Food eaten at lunch | What happened at lunch? | Snacks and drinks | Food eaten at tea | What happened at tea? | Snacks and drinks |
|-----|-----|-----|-----|-----|-----|-----|-----|-----|-----|
| | | | | | | | | | |
| | | | | | | | | | |
| | | | | | | | | | |
| | | | | | | | | | |
| | | | | | | | | | |
| | | | | | | | | | |
| | | | | | | | | | |
| | | | | | | | | | |

those babies that will take only commercially produced puréed baby foods can have gradually increasing amounts of puréed home cooking added.

If the child seems afraid of food or overly fastidious, then encouraging him to touch and play with food without any expectation of eating should reduce tensions and may increase his interest. When children seem to have little idea of how to chew, it can help if the parent demonstrates chewing and biting. Games that encourage the child to develop oral musculature can also help. Examples include: blowing through a straw into water, blowing bubbles, or licking honey off the lips.

In extreme cases of failure to manage solid foods, referral to a speech and language therapist may provide a specialist assessment of oral-motor function.

### Food refusal

At around the age of 9–15 months many children start to refuse food offered to them on a spoon. This is commonly associated with extreme faddiness. This behaviour occurs in about 10% of children, who nearly all manage to thrive, but are a cause of great concern to their parents.[3] This problem may be due to coercive or rushed feeding by the parent at a time when the child is developing a newfound sense of self. The child asserts his autonomy by closing his mouth and turning away and this is when mealtimes can become a battle.

The first step in managing these children is to make a detailed assessment of the problem, including a food diary, and establish that the child is physically well and thriving. This enables the health professional to reassure the parent that the child is growing normally and offer simple practical advice. Most of these children are being offered snacks between meals, usually because the parents are anxious about their nutritional status. The first step is to cut out all food between meals (including sweets, crisps and sugary drinks).

The next step is to offer straightforward advice about meals. These management tips can be given to parents to act as reminders (Box 16.1 can be photocopied and stuck onto the refrigerator).

**BOX 16.1** Management tips for parents with a child who refuses food

> Try not to give your child *anything* between meals that will fill him up or spoil his appetite (this means not just food but also sweets, snacks and sweet drinks).
> At mealtimes, offer a small range of food in small portions.
> Offer food without putting any pressure on the child to eat it.
> Eat with your child if possible.
> Don't offer alternative menus.
> Don't fuss about irrelevancies such as order of courses, finger feeding and messiness.
> Avoid too many drinks at the table.
> Praise the child if any food is eaten.
> Remove food without comment after 20 minutes if he doesn't eat any.
> However little your child eats at a mealtime, try not to give any snacks between meals, or he will get used to obtaining his nourishment this way.

Mealtimes should be stress-free times with clear expectations. Parents should be encouraged to offer meals in a positive manner with encouragement for the child to eat, preferably in a family meal situation. All eating should be given positive praise and attention and any food refusal should be ignored. Food should include choices the child likes and only one new food should be introduced at a time, included with food the child will eat. Any food not eaten should be removed after 20 minutes with no comment at all. Substitute foods should not be offered then or later.

Special mealtimes that make eating fun such as picnics or dolls' tea parties can help children to take more of an interest in food but should not be used too frequently as they can increase the focus on concerns about food.

### Unacceptable mealtime behaviour

The parent may have no concerns about the child's nutritional intake but feel that there are major issues of discipline at meal times. This includes situations when the child refuses to sit at the table. Meals become protracted episodes, or parents alternate between cajoling and force-feeding the child. The child may refuse food offered knowing that the parent will then offer more attractive tastes. In all these situations, the child is controlling the situation and being rewarded with prolonged adult attention (whether it is positive or negative), and other advantages such as more attractive food or extra playing time.

All these problems can be dealt with using simple behavioural techniques such as removing attention for the unwanted behaviour (not eating), and providing encouragement for desired behaviours (sitting at table, eating what is offered). In general terms the parent agrees to make no comment if the child refuses food and to reward acceptable behaviour with praise and attention. It also helps for the parents to model the desired behaviour, by sitting at the table and eating with the child. A reward can be offered if the child behaves well, and it is important to stress that the parent should not reward food refusal by offering more tempting foods.

### BOX 16.2 Case Example

By the age of four years, Laura has become increasingly fussy at home about what she will eat. Her mother, Jasmine, discusses her concerns with her health visitor.

The health visitor soon works out that there are frequent arguments at mealtimes between Laura and her parents about how little she will eat. Laura recently had an episode of diarrhoea and vomiting, since when her appetite seems not to have returned to normal; to compensate for this, both parents have been offering lots of snacks to Laura between meals. Family life is becoming rather fraught.

The health visitor measures Laura's weight and height and plots them on her growth chart, which enables her to reassure Jasmine that Laura has remained on the same centiles.

The health visitor meets with Jasmine and Laura's father Graham. Together the three of them plan a mealtime regime that includes foods that Jasmine's parents know she likes to eat. They agree a regular routine that includes offering copious attention when Laura eats something and ignoring her when she eats nothing. Both parents agree to make no comments about leftover food or mess and not to offer Laura any snacks between meals.

Initially, Jasmine and Graham need a lot of reassurance that Laura is going to eat enough. At first, Laura is adamant she will eat nothing at mealtimes, but with encouragement from the health visitor, Jasmine and Graham manage to be both firm and positive with Laura. A calmer mealtime routine gradually emerges. The health visitor telephones weekly at an agreed time to troubleshoot any problems and monitor progress.

Laura continues to eat a diet with a limited range, but which Jasmine and Graham can see is nutritionally adequate. They agree with the health visitor to continue slowly introducing new foods, but no longer need her support.

### Children with autistic spectrum disorders

Children with autistic spectrum disorders are often very fussy eaters and may need particular understanding with regard to diet. They will often stick to a very limited repertoire of food, eating the same menu day after day. In these circumstances, it may be best not to make any attempt to alter the child's eating pattern, but rather to accept that he has an idiosyncratic attitude to food. Carers may need support to accept this at first, but usually develop a satisfactory diet for the child within the limited repertoire of foods that the child will accept.

It may also be helpful to discuss this with the staff at school who supervise the child's midday meal. Packed lunches may be easier for the child to manage than cooked dinners: staff may need to make some allowances for the content of the lunch box.

### Pica

This is defined as eating substances not normally regarded as food, and should not be confused with mouthing, which is a normal developmental stage. A number of toddlers go through a usually brief phase of experimenting with eating unpleasant substances. Advice on home safety and removal of toxic substances is an important part of child health surveillance at this time. A common point of contact with the primary healthcare team occurs following ingestion of a potentially toxic substance: as well as offering appropriate advice on acute management (often following consultation with the local poisons unit), it is useful to reinforce the home safety message.

The other group who may be affected are older children, usually boys, who gain status amongst their friends by eating disgusting substances. Although this is rarely harmful it can be difficult to prevent. Advice about other ways of handling these challenges may be helpful!

Pica may be associated with developmental delay or iron deficiency, and if old paint is being ingested, there may be a risk of lead poisoning. If the pica seems particularly persistent, these possibilities should be considered.

### Rumination

Rumination is defined as the repeated regurgitation and re-chewing of food without associated gastrointestinal or other medical disorder, such as oesophageal reflux.[4] It is rare but serious, because of its association with failure to thrive. It is often associated with developmental delay, particularly in older children. It can be difficult to distinguish at first from the possetting seen in normal infants, but vomiting may be so frequent and copious as to leave a noxious odour and a demoralised parent. If the symptom persists for longer than a month, and the amount brought up appears sufficient to cause poor growth, a period of observation on a paediatric ward should be requested.

### REFERRAL

Consider assessment by the general practitioner or paediatric referral if the child's weight is below the third centile or there is a fall across centiles: this may need further investigation.

It is tempting to dismiss all behavioural feeding problems as unimportant unless they impair growth. For the parent, a child's refusal to eat as expected may cause endless anguish; and once such habits become established, they can be very difficult to shift. Treatment is more likely to be successful if completed by the age of six years, and ideally before school entry. The earlier a behavioural approach is adopted, along the lines described above, the more likely it is to be successful. In most cases, this can be done by the health visitor. Occasionally, various combinations of paediatric dietician, clinical psychologist and speech and language therapist teams may be necessary. Above the age of six, psychological interventions are less likely to be successful, mainly because feeding habits become more entrenched. Success may however be achieved when the child is old enough to want to change his own diet,[5] or has increased in self-awareness and motivation. Parents sometimes need a lot of reassurance about not intervening too much at this time.

**BOX 16.3** Practice Points about feeding problems

Feeding problems are extremely common in preschool children.

It is essential to plot the child's weight and height on a centile chart.

Food diaries can be helpful in assessment of food intake and carers' behavioural responses.

Simple behavioural programmes, using differential attention for desired and undesired behaviours, can be very effective.

It is worth exploring ways in which meals can be made more fun and enjoyable (rather than a battle or an exercise in calorie-counting).

Early detection and advice during routine child health surveillance can prevent problems developing.

## RESOURCES: BOOKS FOR PARENTS

- Conway R. *Meals without Tears: how to get your child to eat healthily and happily*. London: Prentice Hall Life; 2007.
  This book encourages healthy eating and gives advice on how to help a child develop a healthy attitude to food and how to manage common difficulties parents may face. It encourages a parent to reflect upon her own behaviour and attitudes towards food.
- Karmel A. *Weaning*. London: Dorling Kindersley; 2010.
  This step-by-step guide to weaning provides information on all aspects of weaning including what equipment you need, how to feed your baby and what types of foods to introduce when. There are purée recipes as well as a wide range of easy-to-follow recipes for main meals and puddings.
- Karmel A. *Feeding Your Baby and Toddler*. London: Dorling Kindersley; 2010.
  This is a well-structured, easy-to-read and comprehensive guide on feeding children a healthy, balanced diet and is also packed with recipes. It describes the changing dietary needs of children and how to make food tempting to a child.
- Karmel A. *The Fussy Eaters' Recipe Book: 135 quick, tasty and healthy recipes that your kids will actually eat*. London: Atria Books; 2008.
  Packed with ideas on how to make healthy food fun and tempting, this manual gives tips on how to encourage fussy eaters to get involved in all aspects of food, how to make mealtimes less stressful and how to make eating an enjoyable family experience.

## REFERENCES

1 Butler NR, Golding J, editors. *From Birth to Five: a study of health and behaviour in Britain's five-year-olds*. London: Pergamon Press; 1986.
2 Illingworth RS, Lister J. The critical or sensitive period with specific reference to certain feeding problems in infants and children. *J Paediatr*. 1964 Dec; **65**: 839–48.
3 Richman N, Stevenson J, Graham PJ. *Preschool to School: a behavioural study*. London: Academic Press; 1982.
4 American Psychiatric Association. *Diagnostic and Statistical Manual of Mental Disorders, Version IV*. Washington DC: American Psychiatric Association; 1994.
5 Lask B. Personal communication.

# CHAPTER 17

# Tantrums, aggression and sibling rivalry

## TANTRUMS

Tantrums are a normal feature of development in the preschool years. They are particularly likely to occur when the child is tired, ill, feeling insecure, or stressed in any other way. Unfortunately they can also become a regular pattern for a child who has learnt that tantrums are a means of getting his own way, getting his needs met or getting attention. The parents may then experience an increase in the number or duration or severity of tantrums.

Tantrums become a problem when parents feel that they are too frequent or too intense for them to manage, or when the child is becoming old enough for the parents to say they are worried about the potential harm caused by destructive behaviour.

## ASSESSMENT

Assessment should be specific: examining one or two recent examples, and general: thinking about background factors. There are several options for management, some of which are discussed in a more general way in Chapter 13.

The clearest way of getting relevant details about a recent example is to use the ABC mnemonic – Antecedents, Behaviour and Consequences (*see* Table 17.1). This can also be used for almost any behavioural problem.

**Start with the B (behaviour):** What exactly constitutes a tantrum? How long did it last and what did the child actually do?

**Next establish C (consequences):** Who does what, exactly, during and after a tantrum? Find out how the situation was resolved by the parent. If the parent says she ignores the child, be sure to check on this: exactly what does ignoring consist of?

**Lastly, find out the A (antecedents):** What were the immediate precipitants? As well as a description of what the child was demanding or doing at the time, this might include the parent having a temper outburst themselves, or otherwise behaving unreasonably. Few parents will tell you this spontaneously or early in the consultation, so leave it until after establishing the behaviour and consequences, and specifically ask: 'What exactly were you doing just before he started to shout …?'

**TABLE 17.1** An ABC diary

| Date, time, place | Antecedents | Behaviour | Consequences |
|---|---|---|---|
| Supermarket checkout, Friday, 11 am | Being bored; seeing the sweets on the rack | Screaming, shouting, kicking | I was embarrassed – everyone was watching. I had to give in; then the screaming stopped |
| Friday evening, 7 pm | Not being allowed to go on playing with his trains (because it was bedtime) | Wailing and moaning | I carried him up to bed, got him ready, and read him a story – which distracted him. |
| Saturday morning, 8 am | Not being allowed to have sweets for breakfast | Shouting and screaming | I said he could have some cereal and juice and put these in front of him instead of the sweets. He sulked for a couple of minutes, then ate some cereal, then seemed calmer. |

General assessment should consider, in particular, the following issues.

➤ The **general health** of the child, including pain or other discomfort, and fatigue (usually due to insufficient sleep). Has there been a head injury? (Even apparently minor head injuries can lead to a change in personality and some disinhibition.)

➤ **Delayed language development** will lead the child to be frustrated at not being able to communicate his needs. Check that hearing has been adequately assessed.

➤ The child's **developmental age**. A child with developmental or intellectual delay will be slower to grow out of childish practices, and slower to learn tolerance, adequate communication or postponement of gratification.

➤ **Consistency** of parental discipline. Parents who promise rewards or punishments but find it difficult to follow through are liable to be less effective at instilling trust and discipline. A child with two parents who disagree in front of him, for instance about rewards or consequences for his behaviour, is likely to become confused, but will probably eventually work out a way to stir up the conflict, since this will give him more control over the situation, and he will get away with more.

➤ **Modelling**. A child who has witnessed older siblings or parents having a tantrum is more likely to maintain this behaviour, and less likely to learn alternative ways of resolving frustration or conflict.

➤ Check **medications**. Some can affect behaviour, including most anticonvulsants and some nocturnal sedatives, such as antihistamines.

➤ What about the **mental state of the child**? Children are often much more irritable and difficult to handle when tired or hungry. Is she distressed about bullying or domestic violence? Is she irritable or depressed for some other reason?

➤ *Does the parent have particular stresses* that are making child management more difficult? Are there any mental health issues affecting a carer or close family member? Is there adult substance misuse or domestic violence?

For those who like mnemonics, you can remember this as *the eight 'D's*:
*Discomfort* in the child due to ill health
*Delay* in language
*Developmental* delay
*Discipline* inconsistent or muddled
A *display* of tantrums by others
*Drugs* which may affect behaviour
*Distress* in the child due to internal pressures such as fatigue or hunger, or external pressures such as bullying or abuse
*Distress* in the parent due to external pressures.


## MANAGEMENT
The assessment may throw up some opportunities for advice.
Management can be divided into four broad areas.
➤ *Avoiding provocation or dangerous antecedents* by planning to minimise situations which make the child feel thwarted, or giving the child some distraction *before* this happens.
➤ *Teaching the child alternative strategies.* Children need to have some way of responding to frustration and calming themselves down. One of the reasons tantrums persist in some children is because they have not learnt any other response. It could be helpful to discuss with parents what they think this should be.
➤ *Withdrawing attention* that would reinforce the behaviour (ignoring or time out – *see* Chapter 13 on Behaviour Management).
➤ *Providing positive attention* for all wanted behaviours.

*Avoiding provocation* includes manipulating the environment as much as possible to minimise temptations and frustrations. Examine the antecedents, and you may come up with specific ideas. Some children, for instance, may be particularly helped by forewarning of events known to produce tantrums, such as having to stop a favourite activity, or having to go to bed, for example: 'After this television programme it will be time for your bath'.
*Devise alternative ways of responding to frustration.* If the child does not have a tantrum, what should he do? Discuss this with the parent in relation to the examples of tantrums elicited. If the answer is that he should comply with a parental command, then compliance must be rewarded with labelled praise (praise that specifies exactly what has been done well). A star chart or other reward system can be used for compliance with a particular sort of command, such as getting ready for bed without making a fuss. Effective sorts of command, reward systems, and other methods of improving compliance are discussed also in Chapter 13.

***Withdrawing attention*** is the mainstay of management for many undesired behaviours, tantrums included. The basic principle is that behaviours are maintained by the attention they receive, whether this is positive *or* negative attention, so will be extinguished when that attention is taken away. This is likely to be more effective when attention is given for desired behaviour (which many parents forget to do). There is nothing wrong with the traditional advice to ignore a tantrum; it is just very difficult to put into practice. Simply suggesting it is not enough.

There are two ways to withdraw attention.

➤ The parent can ***remove herself***; the parent can stay in the same place but attend exclusively to something else (ignoring). This can be reassuring for the parent as she stays in the vicinity and thus knows her child is safe. She does need, however, to look busy doing something such as reading a book or carrying out a chore.

➤ The parent can ***remove the child*** to an environment which is entirely non-stimulating (time-out). It is not always possible to leave the child in situ to have their tantrum (for instance, if something is cooking), nor can dangerous behaviours be ignored (such as hurting a baby sibling).

***Positive attention.*** It is also important to develop a positive relationship with the child, for instance by play, and to get into the habit of praising and rewarding whenever possible. Play, praise, rewards, ignoring and time-out are all discussed in more detail in Chapter 13.

## Working with parents

Parents need continuing encouragement to make behavioural techniques work. Frequent appointments and home visits, or regular attendance at a parenting group, may be necessary. A diary, in the form of the above ABC chart, may help.

Many parents are discouraged when trying new techniques of managing a child's behaviour. They find it gets worse, and give up the technique. It is helpful to warn parents that this is to be expected. An undesired behaviour will usually get more frequent before getting less frequent (the so-called '***extinction burst***'). For instance, the first time a parent tries to ignore a tantrum, it is likely to get louder or more desperate.

**BOX 17.1** Case Example

James, aged three years, has a tantrum every time his mother takes him shopping. This is usually in the checkout queue of the supermarket, where there are enticing sweets. He will not stop until his mother gives in and buys him some sweets.

This behaviour could be modified by changing the antecedents (A) in the following ways:

• not taking James shopping
• going to a supermarket that does not have sweets at the checkout

- saying he can have a limited number of sweets, and getting these before the tantrum begins
- distracting him from wanting sweets by buying him something, such as a comic, which is not so bad for his teeth.

The behaviour (B) could be managed by:
- praising James profusely every time he manages the supermarket shop without having an outburst, and possibly backing this up with tangible rewards.

The consequences (C) could be managed by:
- ignoring the tantrum until it stops. This may be impossible if other people in the queue are watching critically (within a supermarket, withdrawing attention can be extremely difficult)
- putting James in time-out just outside the supermarket.

## REFERRAL

When should referral be made? A lot depends on the local service. In a district with well-organised child mental health provision, health visitors should receive regular training in dealing with behavioural problems, which should also provide opportunities for consultation. There will then be very few preschool behaviour problems which require referral. Children with tantrums may need referral when: there are concerns about the underlying mental state of the child; family issues are thought to need detailed discussion; or appropriate behavioural management, with motivated parents, has failed to shift the behaviour. There is no age above which tantrums should be referred; with older children, a lot depends on the associated problems. The older the child, the more entrenched the child's behaviour becomes, so it is more difficult for a change in carer behaviour to elicit a change in child behaviour.

**BOX 17.2** Practice Points for managing tantrums

As well as details of the behaviour, find out about antecedents and consequences (ABC).
Assess possible background factors.
Try some or all of:
- avoiding provocative *antecedents*
- teaching alternative *behaviours*
- withdrawing attention, or other reinforcing *consequences*
- rewarding all wanted behaviours.

Warn parents that things may get worse before they get better.

## AGGRESSION

The causes of aggression are multiple. The following points may be worth remembering.

➤ Aggressive responses can be *learned*. This can be by modelling (for instance, witnessing a violent parent); being rewarded for aggressive behaviours by parents (for instance by a father who believes fighting is the best way to deal with any conflict with peers); or finding that aggression works as a way of resolving conflict.

➤ Aggressive responses are *primitive*, and are likely to be used when the child has no alternative strategies. Therefore they are common in younger children, and those who have not been taught other ways of dealing with provocation. It also means there are opportunities to teach more sociable responses.

➤ Aggressive behaviours are often *an expression of feelings* which may be difficult to express in other ways, for instance anger, irritability, resentment, grief or sadness. Feeling threatened or provoked may also lead to aggression, so that it is a common end-point to a variety of situations.

➤ Aggression is a remarkably *stable* characteristic of behaviour. Once established as a general way of coping, it does not usually go away by itself. Hence reassurance that it will subside, without any other intervention, is likely to be misleading.

## ASSESSMENT

Several factors may contribute to a child's excessive use of aggression as a coping strategy.

Parents may demonstrate aggression in personal relationships in the home and with extended family: rows, harsh physical punishments, verbal threats or domestic violence. Problem-solving may not be a big part of the family culture. There may be few, if any, *role models* for peaceful ways of dealing with conflict, so that the child does not have an opportunity to learn self-restraint or negotiation.

*Media modelling* may also be a factor: violence seen on television news, films or console games.

Aggression may arise out of a combination of *learning* that the best way to respond to a tight situation is with a fight, plus a failure to learn alternative responses, such as walking away, compromising, calming techniques, conciliation or quiet discussion.

Some children may be biologically predisposed to finding these alternative solutions difficult to learn. This does not necessarily mean having a categorical diagnosis. Examples include the following:

➤ being *impulsive*, in other words reacting to provocation without thinking

➤ some children may become more hyperactive or aggressive after certain *foods* (*see* Chapter 44 on Diet and Exercise).[1] Colourings, preservatives and Coca-Cola are common culprits. The mechanism is unknown, but it is not confined to children with an ADHD diagnosis

➤ having a *language disorder*, which may lead to misunderstanding or frustration

➤ having *autistic traits*, which may mean:
  — finding it difficult to imagine what a situation feels like from the point of view of another
  — misinterpreting friendly gestures as unfriendly
  — failing to grasp unspoken rules
  — taking statements literally
  — needing situations to be predictable
  — having difficulty generalising from a solution that works in one situation to other similar situations
➤ having *callous and unemotional traits*, which means lacking empathy, not showing remorse, and not appearing to mind about the consequences on others of your own actions; it seems that such unempathic children are a different group from the children with autistic traits, mentioned in the previous bullet point, who lack a theory of mind[2]
➤ having a *generalised learning difficulty* (*see* Chapter 35), which impairs various skills, including the ability to problem-solve, the ability to adopt solutions suggested by adults, and the capacity to deal with an unfamiliar situation
➤ having *specific literacy difficulties*, which are strongly associated with a variety of behaviour problems, including aggression, probably through several different mechanisms.

Given a parental complaint about a child's aggressive behaviour, it is important to review the *general factors* mentioned under tantrums, such as the child's medical status, mental state and intellectual abilities.

There should always be a specific enquiry about *bullying*: many bullied children retaliate aggressively, and get into trouble for continuing a fight initiated by someone else. Some children, particularly those with autistic traits, may perceive themselves as victims of bullying, even though the surrounding adults do not; such children may overreact to provocation, and are then seen as the main aggressors. The subjective experience of bullying should nevertheless be taken seriously.

The state of the family is also important: is a preferred sibling getting a better deal, is the problem mainly a relationship with a step-parent, or is one of the parents stressed or unwell? *Domestic violence* is a potent progenitor of aggressive behaviour in children, particularly in a son:

➤ he may have witnessed behaviour which he then copies
➤ he may be very angry about suffering physical abuse himself
➤ he may have a genetic predisposition inherited from one or both parents
➤ he may have a host of unresolved feelings about his parents' relationship.

An ABC analysis may be helpful in highlighting unreasonable or unrecognised provocation and unwitting encouragement from others.

In what *contexts* does the aggression mainly occur: school, home or outside? With whom: fellow pupils, siblings, or friends in the community? The management will depend on where the problem is worst.

## MANAGEMENT AND REFERRAL

The assessment may suggest avenues for further assessment or referral, or give opportunities for practical advice. An ABC analysis is likely to highlight opportunities to avoid triggers and generate new consequences. Sibling rivalry is dealt with separately below. Conflict erupting in school may need addressing at least partly within the school context: bullying and specific or general learning difficulty are important to consider. Anger management and self-esteem groups are often available in the school setting. Fights developing in the community may be prevented by the selection of prosocial friends, or limiting unsupervised time outside of the home, but some parents may find this easier than others. Parents may find they can limit opportunities for aggressive behaviours by keeping their children occupied in enjoyable activities, such as after-school clubs, football or martial arts. Rewarding cooperative behaviours with labelled praise or points systems should help to reinforce alternatives to aggressive behaviour. Time-out can be used for younger children as a last resort.

A child with aggressive behaviour should have some intervention sooner rather than later. Aggressive behaviours easily become habitual, and preschool children are much more likely to change their habits. Children with behaviour problems at school should receive help when the problem is first recognised, and not when they are on the verge of permanent exclusion. If help at one service level is not proving productive, *referral* should be made to a higher service level, or for additional services.

**BOX 17.3**  Case Example

Vicki, a 22-year-old single parent, brings her three-year-old son (and only child) Morgan to see her general practitioner, complaining that Morgan will not do anything that she tells him, and that he screams and kicks when he can't get his own way. She is becoming afraid to take him anywhere, so is going out of the house less and less. The general practitioner finds it difficult to focus on the history because of Morgan's behaviour: he rushes from one part of the clinic room to another, knocking things from the desk onto the floor, and throwing out all the toys from the toy bin in the corner.

The general practitioner knows that Vicki had a difficult pregnancy and a prolonged labour, requiring forceps for a slow foetal heart rate. Morgan was a difficult baby to feed, and woke frequently at night. He has had a series of upper respiratory tract infections recorded in his notes, and the general practitioner has also read that he failed his first hearing test but passed his second.

She tries a habitual trick of holding out her arms to Morgan, who responds by coming and standing in front of her. She manages to examine him while talking to him and smiling at him frequently. The examination shows signs of glue ear on both sides, so she explains to Vicki that Morgan's challenging behaviour might be partly due to his having some hearing impairment. She suggests that Vicki will need to be sure that Morgan has heard her before assuming that he is just being naughty. The doctor refers Morgan for a hearing test, and also asks the health visitor to discuss with Vicki strategies for dealing with Morgan's difficult behaviour: their first meeting is two weeks later.

Six weeks later, the general practitioner re-examines Morgan's ear drums, which seem to be quite normal on this occasion. At a follow-up with the health visitor the following week, Vicki reports that she and Morgan are attending a mother and toddler group two afternoons each week, and Morgan is going to a playgroup for three mornings each week. However, his behaviour seems to be no better at home. Vicki is still very concerned that something should be done about Morgan's behaviour. She is tearful and upset and complains of being very tired, not sleeping and always feeling low in mood. She explains that she has tried – as the health visitor advised her – to ignore Morgan when he is being naughty, but has found this very difficult. Vicki also admits that she finds it very hard to play with Morgan, as the health visitor suggested, and does not really know how to play appropriately with him.

The health visitor arranges for Vicki herself to be assessed by the general practitioner: this leads to Vicki accepting a course of antidepressants. The health visitor then refers Vicki to a parenting group at the local children's centre. Vicki attends weekly; as well as discussing behaviour management techniques, she values meeting other parents experiencing similar problems: she finds the group very supportive. The health visitor keeps in regular contact with Vicki and monitors her progress and Morgan's.

Over the next three months, Vicki's mood improves and she learns strategies for dealing with Morgan and his behaviour. Their relationship improves and he becomes less aggressive towards Vicki. He still has tantrums, but Vicki now knows how to deal with these calmly and quickly. She has also made a new friend at the group whom she sees frequently socially.

**BOX 17.4** Practice Points for managing aggression

Discuss examples of the aggressive behaviour.
Do an ABC analysis.
Think what feelings the aggression might be expressing.
Whose behaviour might it be copying?
Are there any concealed difficulties at school, such as bullying or academic frustration?
Explore opportunities for after-school and weekend activities.
Can carers exert more control over choice of friends?
Advise carers to reward alternative behaviours.
For situations that give rise to aggression, encourage problem-solving.
Ask parents to deal with aggression calmly.
For out-of-control aggression, teach the appropriate use of time-out.

**SIBLING RIVALRY**

Think of this from a *developmental perspective*: the birth of a younger sibling is bound to give rise to feelings of jealousy, particularly in the first child, as the older sibling(s) have to share adult attention, and material things such as living space and toys. Grandparents may show excessive interest in the new arrival; parents may be preoccupied or exhausted. There is scope for some preventive work here.

*Before the birth*, children can be involved actively in preparations, given a doll to care for themselves, and made to feel special.

*After the birth*, parents must ensure they are devoting attention to older children as well as the baby. If gifts are bought for the baby, the older child must have presents also. They can involve older children in baby care, such as unfolding nappies, choosing clothes, brushing hair and other safe tasks that can easily be supervised. This gives each older child an active role in the newly enlarged family. When the baby starts smiling, parents can emphasize to an older child that she is smiling at him. A father may sometimes become more distant after the birth of a second child: point out how important his involvement is for all his children.

It is often *later on*, once the baby crawls or walks and breaks or takes toys, that rivalry begins in earnest. Learning how to cope with disagreement is a necessary developmental task, and may be sorely lacking in only children. Positive outcomes include becoming assertive, expressing feelings and learning how to resolve conflict. Mild teasing by an older sibling may not only be a playful way of communicating affection, but also teach coping strategies for more hurtful teasing at school. As conflict becomes more severe, parents have to decide at what level they will not tolerate abuse of younger siblings, whether physical or emotional.

**ASSESSMENT**

Think about factors contributing to conflict between a sibling pair.

➤ Rivalry tends to be greatest between two children of the same sex.
➤ Do the parents have favourites?
➤ Do the parents label one child as the most difficult?
➤ Is the younger child getting more attention because she is more dependent? Older children seldom accept this as an explanation from the parents, but feel they are being short-changed.

**BOX 17.5** Case Example

| | |
|---|---|
| Sarah: | Mummy, Daniel hit me! |
| Daniel: | She started it. She borrowed my game without asking. |
| Mother: | Daniel, don't be cruel to your little sister. |
| Daniel: | You always take her side! |

➤ An older child who is developmentally delayed, or even just academically less able, may resent tremendously a younger one who catches up.

➤ Are the fights between the children a mimicry of fights between the parents, or an overt expression of conflicts the parents think they have kept concealed? Such children may also fight in an attempt to divert their parents from marital problems. They may hope (not necessarily consciously) that their own misbehaviour will force their parents to be more together.

## MANAGEMENT

Research with concealed video cameras has shown that siblings who fight generally fight a great deal less if they think there is no one watching or within earshot.[3] The implication of this is that **ignoring** will work if applied with sufficient persistence. As discussed in Chapter 13, this can be extraordinarily difficult to do effectively. It may sometimes be enough for parents to say simply 'Settle it yourselves'. More often, a parent will have to completely remove herself.

It is particularly important **not to take sides**. Whatever a parent does must be seen as even-handed. For instance, time-out or consequences (*see* Chapter 13) can be used for fights which parents think are excessive, but should be applied equally to both children. Parents should avoid expressing favouritism, and can approach differences in age or skills by emphasizing the particular strengths of each child. They should steer clear of comparisons in which one comes off worse, such as: 'I wish you would keep your room as tidy as your sister', or 'Please try a little harder with your reading – your brother could do this when he was your age'.

Parents can use sibling fights as an opportunity to teach problem-solving. For instance, a parent could show her squabbling children two puppets who are fighting over a toy, or say that one wants to use a toy that the other won't let him have. She could then guide her children in generating possible solutions to the dilemma, and discuss the consequences of each solution. With school-age children, a family meeting can be a useful opportunity to explore solutions to conflicts between two family members. This could be at a regular time each week.

## WHEN TO REFER

Sibling quarrels are a normal and healthy phenomenon. Most parents who present them as a problem can be helped to see them as a developmental challenge, and as an opportunity for learning interpersonal skills, as suggested above. In some cases, fights between siblings may be part of a broader behavioural problem, in which case referral to specialist CAMHS may be justified. In other cases, children may be at risk of significant abuse from their siblings, in which case social services should be involved. A further possibility is that difficulties in the parents' relationship are at the heart of the problem, in which case relationship counselling could be suggested.

**BOX 17.6** Practice Points for managing sibling rivalry

Describe how a certain amount of quarrelling develops skills.

How did the problem develop?

Is there a favourite?

Are there differences in ability?

Is there marital conflict?

How are the parents dealing with the sibling conflicts? Does this calm or fan the flames?

Advise ignoring if no one is coming to harm.

Is there scope for problem-solving when things are calm?

Advise time-out or consequences if someone is getting hurt.

## RESOURCES

### Books and websites for parents on behaviour management

- There is a list of such books and websites at the end of Chapter 13.

### Books for children on temper

- Oram H, Kitamura S. *Angry Arthur*. London: Andersen Press; 2008.
  This book is a vivid pictorial description of a three year old's tantrum.
- Sendak M. *Where the Wild Things Are*. London: Red Fox; 2000.
  This is the classic story of a child's journey to fantasy land, where his feelings are embodied.

### Books for children on sibling rivalry

- Browne A. *The Tunnel*. London: Walker Books; 2008.
  This story is for children of four to eight years. A brother and sister who are always fighting discover that their affection for each other is stronger than they thought.
- Flack M. *Angus and the Cat*. London: Farrar, Straus & Giroux; 1997.
  Angus the dog is jealous of the cat when he first discovers that he's not an 'only child' anymore.

### BOOKS FOR PARENTS ON SIBLING RIVALRY

- Faber A, Mazlish E, Coe KA. *Siblings Without Rivalry: how to help your children live together so you can live too (how to help your child)*. London: Piccadilly Press; 1999.
  This book is for parents who would like to think about and improve relationships between their children, partly through understanding each child's point of view.
- Parker J, Stimpson J. *Raising Happy Brothers and Sisters: helping our children enjoy life together, from birth onwards*. London: Mobius; 2004.
  This book includes parental and professional perspectives on how to improve relationships within families of all shapes and sizes.

## REFERENCES

1 McCann D, Barrett A, Cooper A, *et al*. Food additives and hyperactive behaviour in 3-year-old and 8/9-year-old children in the community: a randomised, double-blinded, placebo-controlled trial. *Lancet*. 2007; **370**(9598): 1560–7.

2 Jones AP, Happé FGE, Gilbert F, *et al*. Feeling, caring, knowing: different types of empathy deficit in boys with psychopathic tendencies and autism spectrum disorder. *J Child Psychol Psychiatry*. 2010; **51**(11): 1188–97.

3 Dadds MR. Personal communication.

# CHAPTER 18

# Breath-holding

## INTRODUCTION

There are two sorts of breath-holding attacks: blue and white. Most start between six and 18 months and disappear by six years.

*Blue (cyanotic) spells* are found in babies and toddlers and are common, affecting up to 5% of children. They appear to run in families. A typical blue spell is precipitated by frustration, rage or pain. This may begin with what is otherwise a typical temper tantrum in which the yelling and crying leads to the ultimate expression of frustration: a determined closure of the back of the throat, which blocks further breathing – so that no air is now getting into the lungs. This sounds serious, but is actually self-limiting, because the child becomes blue (cyanosed) and then loses consciousness, which stops her keeping her throat closed, and so allows breathing to start again. The child may become rigid, and occasionally have a few clonic movements (to-and-fro jerky movements of the limbs of the sort that are seen in epileptic fits). Recovery is swift and complete. The differences from epilepsy are: a clear precipitant (usually being thwarted), the occurrence of forceful crying and then cyanosis before loss of consciousness, and the absence of drowsiness after the episode.

*White (pallid) spells* are different, and likely to be more concerning. Following surprise, pain or mild injury – such as bumping the head in a fall while learning to walk, the first experience of an adult bath, or a new taste – the child falls limp and stops breathing. Crying and yelling do not usually come before the breath-holding, the last breath is not necessarily an out-breath, and the child is usually white rather than blue. However, the heart rate may slow down, and the lack of oxygen may lead to a seizure that is indistinguishable from epilepsy. Recovery is swift and uneventful, except when there is a seizure, in which case there may be some drowsiness after the episode. The risk of epilepsy is no greater than in the general population, but there is a tendency when older to faint in response to pain or surprise.

Breath-holding attacks, whether blue or white, can be very frightening for most parents, particularly those who have never seen one before. To see your own child stop breathing, whatever the cause, will understandably and naturally generate anxiety: if it doesn't, then that might in itself be a concern for the professional.

## ASSESSMENT, MANAGEMENT AND REFERRAL

Breath-holding attacks can be diagnosed by history alone. In view of the likely anxiety generated by any breath-holding episode, the assessment process and any intervention should be preceded by active listening. Otherwise, carers may perceive you as not understanding how serious it seems to them. Only once they have experienced empathy are they likely to be able to deal with the child in a dispassionate way.

## REFERRAL

*All* children with white attacks and any child whose blue attacks have an atypical history should be referred to a paediatrician. Referral to a paediatrician should also be made in the presence of other paediatric conditions such as developmental delay, or any other potential cause of seizures. A child with blue spells usually also has a history of behavioural issues such as tantrums, oppositional behaviour or at least a determination to get his own way. The blue spell often occurs as the climax of such behaviour. If there is no clear link to this sort of behaviour, then a general practitioner and/or paediatrician should review the child.

*Note:* What follows is only about *blue* breath-holding (as all children with a white attack should be referred).

## PSYCHOEDUCATION

An adequate explanation of blue breath-holding should precede any discussion of management. Parents usually want to know whether it is dangerous (it is not: brain damage does not occur); whether it is epilepsy (it is clearest to say no); and whether it may turn into persistent seizures (it does not). Children are likely to grow out of blue breath-holding attacks long before they grow out of tantrums. Carers may also ask for advice on how to terminate attacks when they occur.

## INTERVENTIONS

The intervention that works best is active ignoring. As with the management of tantrums (*see* Chapter 17), the child should be given minimal or no attention, so as not to reinforce the breath-holding behaviour. The carer(s) should be encouraged to deal with the child calmly after the attack, with the minimum of fuss and no punishment, and to continue whatever activity was taking place before. It may also be worth emphasising what should be obvious to some parents – that the child should be protected from harm during the brief spell of unconsciousness. Also as with tantrums, it is usually helpful to identify triggers so that these can be avoided, and to use distraction (at an early stage) if possible: diverting the child to something he wants to do, to take his mind off his frustration. Some children can be helped to express their frustration in an alternative way: playing with drums, doing an extra-colourful drawing or running around outside for a while are possible examples.

Once they are convinced that the child will come to no harm, parents usually find ignoring breath-holding attacks is straightforward and effective. Parental anxiety or panic may lead to overprotectiveness and giving in to the breath-holding spells, which may make it difficult for parents to be firm and ignore effectively. In this case, parents may benefit from advice and support from their health visitor or community school nurse. If this fails to reassure them, an assessment by a general practitioner may be necessary, and finally a paediatric referral.

**BOX 18.1** Practice Points for blue breath-holding attacks

Take a careful history.

If the history is unclear or if parental reassurance is difficult, a general practitioner review may be necessary, possibly followed by a paediatric referral.

If there is a clear history of a behavioural build-up to breath-holding:

- listen to the carer's anxieties
- develop an understanding of what triggers the behaviour
- explain that the condition is common and causes no long-term damage
- ensure parents will keep the child safe during any period of unconsciousness
- ask carers to avoid triggers if possible
- recommend active ignoring
- advise against giving in to what is effectively a tantrum
- discuss possible alternative ways for the child to express his frustration.

## RESOURCES

- www.healthvisitors.com
- www.kidsbehaviour.co.uk

# CHAPTER 19

# Headbanging and body-rocking

## INTRODUCTION

Carers may seek advice about headbanging and body-rocking from professionals in Tier 1 and Tier 2. They will have noticed a repetitive motion that apparently occurs for no reason. It is usually seen when the child is relaxing, drowsy or going off to sleep. It can be both disconcerting and annoying to other members of the family if the child carries out this behaviour whilst, for example, sitting on the sofa with them. It can also be very noisy. The child himself is completely unfazed and may well be unaware of the behaviour. Carers often worry that it is a sign of a significant mental health problem in the child or that it could cause brain damage and therefore seek reassurance.

Headbanging and body-rocking are examples of **stereotypies** – spontaneous repetitive movement patterns that occur in young children, apparently without purpose. The child rhythmically moves his head or torso in a back-and-forth motion. These behaviours happen in normal children, although they are commoner in children with a learning disability or autistic spectrum disorder. In normal children, the peak age of onset for both behaviours is about nine months. By the age of 3–6 years, motor stereotypies occur in 3–4% of normal children, while roughly 25% for thumb-sucking and nail-biting.[1] Other behaviours seen in normal children include hair-twisting and face-pulling.[2]

## ASSESSMENT, MANAGEMENT AND REFERRAL

When assessing this problem it is reassuring for carers if you *take a history* of the problem, identifying **when and where it occurs**. From the history, you may well discover that the parent has a fear that the child will harm himself, or a belief that the behaviour is a sign of abnormal development. It is therefore worth carrying out a **developmental check** and referring for a paediatric assessment if any concerns are noted. It is also worth considering whether there may be any **physical problem** that could cause long-term pain such as a chronic ear infection. For some children, particularly those with some other source of pain or with learning difficulties, the pain of the contact with a hard surface may serve a valuable function. Some children may cause a bald patch on whichever part of the head is regularly banged or rubbed. Otherwise, it is unlikely that any significant harm will ensue.

A detailed description of the ***antecedents and consequences*** of what the child does should distinguish those children who headbang when their wishes are thwarted, in which case the behaviour may be viewed as part of a tantrum and treated accordingly, usually by active ignoring (this may or may not involve an ABC chart – *see* Chapter 17). If the behaviour occurs every time the carer says 'no' to the child, giving in to the headbanging will tend to increase it. Usually the child's behaviour will stop after a period of consistent and persistent ignoring.

If there are no developmental, health or other behavioural concerns, then carers can be reassured that this behaviour is common and that the child will probably grow out of it over time,[3] with or without specific treatment, although some adults do continue to rock to sleep or have repetitive habits.

If ***further management*** is required, minimal attention and intervention are usually the best strategy. Any form of attention is likely to maintain the behaviour. Carers should therefore be supported in ignoring such stereotypies. Some parents will find it very hard to ignore a child hitting his head or body against a hard surface – in which case basic safety measures should be introduced. The parent can, for instance, move the child to a soft area such as a sofa or a corner of the room covered with cushions, without mentioning the behaviour itself. There is however no guarantee that the child will stay there! Distracting the child onto alternative and incompatible activities may also work, but it may be counterproductive to distract a child as he goes off to sleep (*see* also Chapter 13 on Behavioural Management for more on ignoring and distraction).

The noise of such behaviours, especially headbanging, may be very irksome to some carers, particularly if they or other children in the family are trying to get to sleep. Neighbours on the other side of a party wall may complain. Such parents may therefore require additional professional support to use ignoring or distraction effectively. A rehearsal of how to explain the situation to the neighbours may help, as may common-sense measures such as moving the bed to a different wall.

If the behaviour persists despite the above measures, and carers remain concerned, then referral should be discussed. Children with stereotypies should be referred to a community paediatrician if it is mainly further assessment that is required. If it is more detailed treatment that is required, then children with developmental disorders may benefit from a CAMHS learning disability service, if available; and others may benefit from referral to generic specialist CAMHS.

**BOX 19.1** Case Example

Heera attends the health visitor's drop-in clinic with concerns about Asha, aged three years, who rocks as she goes off to sleep. It has become worse over time and is now occurring every night for about 45 minutes, being severe enough to make Asha's bedhead knock against the wall. This has led to some complaints from the neighbours.

The health visitor discusses Asha's development with Heera: there are no other concerns. Asha has started nursery school, where she has settled well; there are no other worries at home.

The health visitor reassures Heera that the behaviour does not indicate some significant underlying problem. They then discuss moving the bed away from the wall so that the neighbours will not be disturbed. They agree that Heera and her husband should ignore the rocking from now on.

The health visitor does a follow-up visit a month later. Asha has continued to rock herself to sleep. Heera has decided to swap the bedrooms in the house around so that Asha's bed is now on an outside wall and not bothering the neighbours anymore.

Heera is by this time feeling less concerned about the rocking. It continues for a further 18 months, gradually reducing in severity over time.

**BOX 19.2** Practice Points for stereotypies

Are there any concerns about development? If so, refer to a community paediatrician.
Are there any concerns about health? If so, refer to an acute or community paediatrician.
Are the behaviours part of other behaviour problems, such as tantrums? If so, treat the tantrums.
What harm is the behaviour causing? Minimise the harm.
What bother is the behaviour causing? Minimise the bother.
Can parents be reassured sufficiently to practice ignoring?
If so, persevere with ignoring and distraction.
If not, discuss with carers whether to refer to a community paediatrician, the local CAMHS learning disability service if there is one, or the local generic CAMHS.

## RESOURCES

- www.healthvisitors.com
- www.kidsbehaviour.co.uk

## REFERENCES

1 Foster LG. Nervous habits and stereotyped behaviors in preschool children. *J Am Acad Child Adolesc Psychiatry.* 1998; **37**(7): 711–7.
2 Troster H. Prevalence and functions of stereotyped behaviors in non-handicapped children in residential care. *J Abnorm Child Psychol.* 1994; **22**(1): 79–97.
3 Abe K, Oda N, Amatomi M. Natural history and predictive significance of head-banging, head-rolling and breath-holding spells. *Dev Med Child Neurol.* 1984; **26**(5): 644–8.

# PART 4

# Middle childhood

# CHAPTER 20

# Anxiety, worry, fears and phobias

## INTRODUCTION

Anxiety is a combination of emotions, bodily sensations and thoughts that form a continuum from normal to abnormal. There is no clear cut-off point separating normal from abnormal anxiety. A certain amount of anxiety may actually improve performance, but as shown in Figure 20.1, increasing anxiety will eventually lead to decreased performance. Anxiety is *abnormal* when it affects the child's ability to participate in expected age-appropriate social or academic activities – in other words, when it causes significant impairment.

### Definitions

Pathological anxiety may be ***generalised*** (present for much of the time in most situations) or ***specific*** (related to a single object or situation) – when it may be called a ***phobia*** (which is merely the Latin word for fear). Examples include spider phobia, dog phobia and social phobia. In many cases, the phobia may have an experiential origin: for instance being approached by a scary, growling dog (of which the child may be justly scared), or being bullied by peers. In other cases, the precipitating factors may be unclear.

Anxiety may occur continuously or in discrete bursts, such as ***panic attacks***. These are clusters of physiological symptoms, emotions and thoughts. A prominent part is usually played by arousal of the autonomic (involuntary) nervous system, and the resulting hormonal and other changes (*see* Table 20.1), which can be neatly summed up in the phrase 'fight or flight reaction', as it includes features of this normal hunter-gatherer response to being confronted by a dangerous beast such as a tiger. In present-day life, there may be various triggers (not usually tigers), and the response could perhaps more comprehensively be called 'fight, flight or freeze'. Associated thoughts include a strong desire to escape from or avoid the trigger or situation leading to the panic attack, and an underlying ***fear*** – which is also a strong emotion. The underlying fear is typically something like:
- a fear of making a fool of oneself (or of being thought uncool)
- a fear of dying
- a fear of collapsing or fainting
- a fear of being sick
- a fear of going mad.

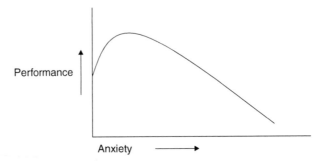

**FIGURE 20.1** The relationship between increasing anxiety and success in performance

**TABLE 20.1** Physiological (autonomic) features of a panic attack

| All over the body | In a central part of the body | Affecting the body's peripheries |
| --- | --- | --- |
| Dizziness | A choking or smothered feeling | Going pale |
| Feeling faint | Shortness of breath, usually due to breathing too fast – hyperventilation | A dry mouth |
| Feeling light-headed, unsteady or on the verge of collapse | Pounding heart – palpitations | Sweating |
| Feeling cold or hot all over (sometimes both) | Chest pain or discomfort | Shaking limbs – tremor |
| | Butterflies in the tummy | Pins and needles – paraesthesiae |
| | Nausea | |

The physiological (autonomic) symptoms are often misinterpreted as confirmation of this underlying fear, leading to further anxious thoughts and then worsening physiological symptoms in a vicious spiral.

### Features of anxiety

Anxiety in children can manifest itself in a number of ways.

➤ *Cognitive*
  - *Worry* is the cognitive part of anxiety: thoughts about what might happen that may be repetitive or go round in circles (also called *ruminations* – which may occur also in depression). Younger children or those with learning difficulties may find it hard to put these into words.
  - Children are likely to lack the *self-reflective capacity* to see their emotions and the resulting behaviours as a problem: they are more likely to see the dog or the bullies or the teachers as the problem.

- Fears, as discussed under panic attacks, may have *a cognitive and an emotional component*. The cognitive component is the belief or prediction that something bad is going to happen.
- The cognitive component may however be *difficult to access* in a child of any developmental age. Many children are unaware of their anxious thoughts or worries or at least unable to report them. This may occur particularly with panic symptoms: the child's focus is likely to on the concrete physical symptoms rather than on what was going through her mind just before the panic kicked in.

➤ *Emotional*
- The emotional component of fear is the feeling of dread or some such, which most children would find difficult to put into words.
- Children may be able to say they are scared or worried without being able to explain further.

➤ *Behavioural*. An anxious child may be:
- clingy and reluctant to leave her parent
- avoidant of new situations
- restless or hyperactive
- more obsessional than usual
- socially withdrawn
- reluctant to leave her home
- reluctant to participate in activities she used to enjoy
- slow to get to sleep
- liable to eat less or eat more
- not apparently anxious, particularly if she has successfully avoided the anxiety-provoking situation: for instance, a school-refusing child often seems very calm and well once she is clear that she can successfully avoid school.

➤ *Somatic*. Children may have:
- the sort of autonomic bodily changes described in Table 20.1 above
- vaguer symptoms such as tummy aches or headaches, which may present to general practitioners or paediatricians without any overt signs of anxiety or worry (*see* Chapter 40 on Recurrent Abdominal Pain and Chapter 41 on Physical Presentations of Emotional Distress); such children could be described as being 'sick with worry'.

It is not always obvious to parents or professionals that these behavioural or somatic symptoms are a reflection of anxiety or worry – particularly if alternative explanations are easier to accept. If a child looks pale, a parent is more likely to assume that a doctor is needed – rather than a child mental health professional.

## A developmental perspective

As a child develops, the things that frighten her change. As a young infant, it may be loud noises or bumping into things that generate a fearful reaction, shown by the startle response or bursting into tears. Fear of strangers starts at about nine months. *Separation anxiety* starts at about the same time and should subside gradually by four to five years. It is shown by distress when an attachment figure leaves and clinginess when it looks as if the carer is about to leave: some children follow the carer around everywhere. These behaviours are more marked when there is an insecure attachment, and more apparent in unfamiliar circumstances, or when the child is hungry, tired or unwell.

Isolated fears are common in young children: of the dark, of monsters, or of strange toilets. Such fears become problematic phobias only if they cause excessive distress or avoidance. For instance, most people are justifiably apprehensive of wasps, but a child who refuses to go in the garden at all during the summer for fear of being stung by a wasp could be said to suffer from a wasp phobia.

As a child becomes older, she becomes more concerned about her appearance, performance and what others think of her. Whether these normal concerns develop into problematic anxiety is likely to be influenced by the determinants of the child's views about herself, including: peers, parents, other respected adults and the media. For example, a child's anxieties about her appearance may be exacerbated by name-calling or wanting to be like (but fearing she is not at all like) widespread pictures of a favourite media star. A child's anxieties about her own academic success at school may be prompted by (thinking she does not live up to) parental expectations or the standards set by teachers.

Any anxiety that arises may be reduced or augmented by others around the child. Sometimes, a child's anxiety may have a powerful impact on other family members. Members of the family may inadvertently reinforce the anxiety, for instance by:

➤ repeatedly offering **reassurance** – this is usually intended to make the child feel better, but may paradoxically reinforce and maintain the child's expressions of anxiety
➤ colluding with avoidant behaviours – avoidance also tends to reinforce anxiety, by allowing the anxiety not to be felt, and becoming self-perpetuating if left unchallenged; an example could be avoiding a family social activity due to one child's phobia
➤ paying anxious attention to physiological symptoms.

In some cases, a child's anxiety reflects parental anxiety, most commonly maternal anxiety, agoraphobia or depression.

The authors' clinical experience suggests that in the under-18s, presentations of phobia or panic attack are commoner than presentations of generalised anxiety. This may be partly because symptoms of anxiety in adolescents are commonly combined with symptoms of depression (*see* Chapter 26), and the diagnosis of depression tends to take precedence, because of its inherently greater risks.

## ASSESSMENT

Taking into account the framework detailed above, there are a number of questions to consider.

➤ What is the child afraid of?
➤ Would you expect the circumstances to make any reasonable person anxious (for instance, following a burglary in the home or a murder in the next street)?

➤ Considering the developmental age of the child, are the fears or anxiety age-appropriate? For instance, a four year-old who starts primary school, finds it difficult to fit in, and then freezes on stage during a school play should not be regarded as in any way abnormal.

➤ How does the anxiety show itself?

➤ Is the anxiety causing the child any distress, or interfering with her functioning?

➤ Ask the child to rate her anxiety from zero to 10 (10 being the worst).

➤ How do others react to the way the child shows her anxiety?
  — How are other family members responding to it?
  — Are they inadvertently reinforcing the anxiety, either by giving in to it, or repeatedly offering reassurance?
  — Are they helping the child manage it effectively by insisting that she follows through with feared tasks, such as getting to school or staying in her bedroom on her own?
  — Are staff at school helping the child become less anxious, or inadvertently reinforcing the anxious behaviour?

➤ For panic attacks, it is important to enquire about the underlying fear, which is sometimes difficult to uncover (it may be too frightening even to think about).

➤ Are there symptoms of depression as well as anxiety?

➤ Have there been any recent significant family or individual events? Examples include domestic violence, a road traffic accident or a family member being mugged. Sometimes the recent event may seem relatively trivial, but may echo an event much longer ago of far greater emotional salience (for instance, the recent death and funeral of an unknown great-uncle may echo the death several years ago of a beloved grandparent).

## MANAGEMENT

*Age-appropriate fears* require an explanation to carers that they need not worry – in fact they need actively to ignore the child's behaviour. This may be difficult for some carers for whom the child's fears awaken their own anxiety; in which case the carer may need help to master this independently from the child.

### Out-of-proportion anxiety that causes significant impairment

In an effort to reduce the child's distress, parents may give in to the child's fears by offering frequent reassurance or supporting avoidance tactics. Both tactics are likely to reinforce and maintain the anxiety. Reassurance should therefore be limited to only one reassuring statement, followed by distracting the child onto something other than reassurance-seeking behaviour. Confronting the subject of the avoidance may be more of a challenge, and may need to be introduced in a graded fashion; examples include:

➤ for a child with a dog phobia – going for a walk in a park where there may be dogs

➤ for a child with social phobia – meeting new people

➤ for a child with panic attacks – confronting known triggers

➤ for a child with separation anxiety – going to sleep alone (*see* Chapter 36 on Sleep Problems)
➤ for a child with school refusal – going to school at the normal time for the whole day (*see* Chapter 21 on School Refusal).

The dilemma for parents is that confronting the source of the anxiety may initially make all the symptoms a great deal worse. This is analogous to the 'extinction burst' seen in children when an undesirable behaviour is first ignored, but may be more difficult to manage. The child's distress may increase in all sorts of ways: tears or tummy aches are two simple examples. Such distress can make it extremely difficult for parents to be firm. Professionals need to be tolerant and understanding of the emotional impact on any parent of the child's attempts to maintain avoidance as her preferred strategy.

Parents and children may find books or websites a source of helpful advice: some examples are given under 'Sources of Information' below. Many areas have book-lending or book prescription schemes.

### Cognitive-behavioural techniques for anxiety

Cognitive-behavioural approaches are useful in reducing the child's anxiety and improving her functioning. The main components are as follows, and tend to be more successful when at least one parent is actively involved, as well as the child.

➤ *Psychoeducation* involves explaining to the child and her parents the nature of anxiety, its causes and the factors that maintain it. This should include:
  — an explanation of the continuum between anxiety that is appropriate for age and circumstances and anxiety that is out-of-proportion and causes impairment
  — the physiological, behavioural, emotional and cognitive aspects of anxiety
  — how treatment addresses the different components of anxiety.
➤ *Cognitive restructuring* involves getting the child to identify his anxious thoughts and find other less anxiety-provoking ways of looking at the situation. Anxiety will lead most people to overestimate both the likelihood of something unpleasant happening and the possible consequences of this.
  — Help the child identify her anxious thoughts.
  — Link these with feelings, bodily sensations and behaviours.
  — Explore any vicious circles generated, for instance by interpreting bodily symptoms as an indication of something awful about to happen.
  — Re-rate the chances of feared outcomes actually happening.
  — Find ways of reducing anxiety and feeling calmer. This could include breathing exercises, relaxation techniques or calming thoughts. They may be difficult to do once anxiety builds up, in which case writing them on a cue card may help.
  — Ensure the child praises herself for any success experience, and that parents also praise her.
➤ *Graded exposure* involves getting the child gradually to face the thing(s) she is scared of or avoiding, in a step-wise process (like going up a ladder), so that

any changes are small and increases in anxiety are tolerable. It is important to predict that the child will feel uncomfortable when facing things she is scared of. The task is to learn to manage the fearful feelings, bodily sensations and strong urges to return to avoidance. If she gives in before some progress has been made, then anxiety and avoidance may win.

— The first step is to create a list of feared situations or things and then rank them in order of how difficult they will probably be to face – a **graded hierarchy**. This can be done by the child and the professional, plus or minus a parent.

— Beginning with the least challenging, these are then tackled in turn at a rate that the child can manage. It is important for the child to succeed and to be able to manage the task set, but also for the task to generate some anxiety, so that she has an experience of coping with this stress. For example, a child afraid of spiders may be exposed to pictures of spiders first, then a small plastic one, then a small real one, then gradually larger ones until she feels comfortable and able to manage any anxiety generated.

— The more a child exposes herself to the feared situation, the more the anxiety lessens. This can be illustrated by drawing a simple graph with a brief explanation as shown below.

— Encourage the child and her parents to practice between sessions by setting a homework task (though calling it homework may not have the most positive associations!). Progress can be reviewed at the next session before moving on up the hierarchy.

➤ Encourage **parents** to support the child's progress as much as possible, for instance by encouraging courageous behaviours, praising success and confronting avoidance. Parents need to beware of accidentally reinforcing a child's anxious behaviour by giving in to her demands (for instance when wining or crying) or providing excessive reassurance. Some timely reassurance about

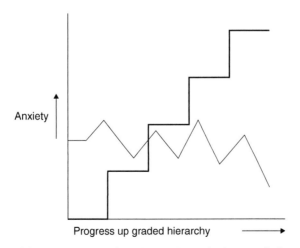

**FIGURE 20.2** Possible time course of anxiety ratings during graded exposure

the child's ability to handle the situation can be helpful, but the child should not become dependent on parental reassurance to confirm that the situation is safe and that she can cope with it: she should learn this through her own experience.

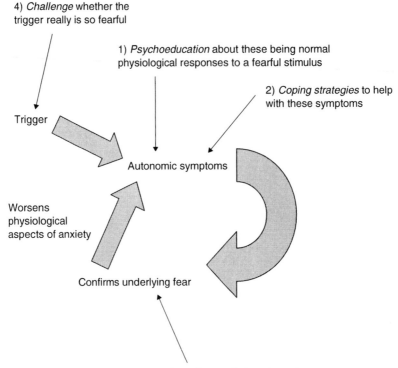

4) *Challenge* whether the trigger really is so fearful

1) *Psychoeducation* about these being normal physiological responses to a fearful stimulus

2) *Coping strategies* to help with these symptoms

Trigger

Autonomic symptoms

Worsens physiological aspects of anxiety

Confirms underlying fear

3) *Ratings* of whether the underlying fear really is going to happen

**FIGURE 20.3** Intervention points in a panic attack

➤ Similar techniques can be used in the management of ***panic attacks***. Identifying the thoughts involved can be a way of tackling the vicious circle shown in Figure 20.3. The autonomic symptoms shown in Table 20.1 are commonly misinterpreted as evidence that the underlying fear is true ('I really *am* going to die').
  — Psychoeducation can emphasise that these are part of the normal fight-or-flight response, and do not indicate an impending heart attack or the onset of insanity.
  — Coping strategies such as measured breathing or relaxation techniques can help reduce the severity of the symptoms.
  — Ratings can help the child realise that the underlying fear is not an inevitable consequence of these physiological symptoms.
  — Lastly, the implications of the trigger fear can be challenged.
➤ An alternative to graded exposure is ***flooding***, which means exposing to a whole situation in one go. For many children and their families, this is simply too

scary to contemplate, but it does seem to be more effective for a few children. It is likely to require prolonged and intensive support from a professional or an adult in the family who is not going to give in. It usually requires sustained field work, so cannot generally be fitted in to an hour's appointment in the clinic.

**BOX 20.1** Case Example

Jodie, a 16-year-old girl, asks to see her community school nurse after experiencing panic attacks. These happen mainly before coming into school or attending assemblies, and sometimes during group social activities. The attacks have recently become more severe and she rates them at eight out of 10 (10 being the worst she can imagine them being). She has started attending the school sick room frequently, which has been concerning the school's welfare assistant.

Jodie cannot think of any specific reasons for her sudden onset of symptoms, but says she has never liked assemblies or large crowds of people. She is due to take her GCSEs in a few months and admits that she is finding the impending exams quite a strain; she has been studying hard at home. As she goes into detail, Jodie becomes tearful and confides that she wonders at times if she is going mad or having a nervous breakdown.

The community school nurse arranges to see Jodie for some further appointments to discuss Jodie's anxiety and how she is dealing with it. She reassures Jodie that she is not going mad and that her symptoms are probably due to her anxiety about GCSEs.

The community school nurse meets with Jodie for six sessions. She educates Jodie about the nature of anxiety and the physiological symptoms she is experiencing. This helps to demystify the situation for Jodie, who then feels more confident to work on the things causing the panic attacks. They discuss specific management strategies including a graded reintroduction to the assemblies: this involves initially sitting at the edge of the hall and then gradually moving further into the room to sit with supportive friends. They take a similar approach to help Jodie get back into group social situations. The community school nurse helps Jodie work on some general management strategies for anxiety, including relaxation techniques, positive thinking and the use of distraction. They discuss study skills and strategies for improving sleep onset, including ways of reducing anxiety at bedtime.

Jodie gives the community school nurse permission to discuss her recent difficulties with key school staff. This leads to Jodie's form tutor offering her some extra individual support with prioritising and planning her course work and revision.

Over the course of the sessions, Jodie's panic attacks reduce, and she reports feeling better able to manage things generally. She stops having regular sessions with the community school nurse, who says she will be available if Jodie needs to contact her during the examination period. Jodie comes once to the drop-in clinic, mainly to say that she feels she is doing better with her exams then she thought she would.

### Medication

With mild to moderate anxiety there is usually no need for medication although young people may want to discuss its use – and may initially request it. A clear explanation of the use of behavioural techniques and their benefits will usually suffice and help them to engage in this sort of treatment, reducing their wish (or parental wishes) for medication.

In some circumstances, young people with severe anxiety may benefit from medication, preferably combined with some psychological intervention. In these cases, referral to specialist CAMHS is indicated for advice on the advantages and disadvantages of medication.

### REFERRAL

Age-appropriate fears should be dealt with by explaining their normality. Simple phobias as in the case example in Box 20.2 could be managed at Tier 1. Panic attacks as in the case example in Box 20.1 are likely to require cognitive-behavioural techniques, which should be available at Tier 2. More complex entrenched problems may require a referral to a specialist CAMHS service.

**BOX 20.2** Case Example

> Kiran, an eight-year-old boy, is brought to his general practitioner by his mother, Mariam, with a complaint that he is unreasonably afraid of cats. This problem has come to a head because yesterday Kiran saw a cat on the pavement, broke away from his mother's hand and ran into the road to get away from the animal. Mariam described how he had screamed and been trembling with fear.
>
> The general practitioner asks about the duration and origin of the symptoms. They have been building up over some months, but Mariam and Kiran cannot identify a specific trigger episode. The general practitioner tells Mariam that something can definitely be done about Kiran's cat phobia, and he refers the family to the primary mental health worker attached to the practice.
>
> At a practice meeting four weeks later, the primary mental health worker describes her progress with the family. Initially, Kiran and Mariam were helped to devise a graded hierarchy of exposure to cats. The bottom step of this consisted of looking at pictures of cats together. The next step involved getting Kiran's brother and sister to pretend to be cats. The next step was looking at cats through a window of the family home; and the next involved a visit to the local pet shop to look closely at a cat through the window. Further planned steps will eventually include encouraging Kiran to enter the same room as someone holding a cat, then moving on to stroking a cat while someone else holds it, with the aim of finally holding a cat himself. The primary mental health worker has not detected an origin or underlying cause to Kiran's cat phobia.

**BOX 20.3** Practice Points about anxiety

Components of anxiety include cognitive, emotional, behavioural and somatic elements.

Anxiety may be generalised or specific. Specific anxiety includes phobias (of objects or situations) and panic attacks.

Assessment should include detailed enquiry about physical sensations, thoughts and feared consequences.

The treatment of choice is usually cognitive-behavioural therapy. It involves facing up to feared situations and overcoming the surges in anxiety that this will produce.

Success is likely to be enhanced by support from parents or close friends.

Medication is not recommended as a first option, or as the only treatment, but may occasionally be of some value for symptomatic relief.

## RESOURCES

- Box 20.4 gives an example of a leaflet that can be handed out to parents. Information about other resources follows.

**BOX 20.4** A handout on anxiety management for the parents of young people

When a child is anxious she tends to seek a lot of reassurance from the adults around her. She may also try to get the household routines changed in order to minimise her anxiety. This may involve, for instance, refusing to go to school, not going out with friends or avoiding family gatherings.

**The young person is trying to control her anxiety by controlling the world around her.** Unfortunately, the more she does this, the more anxious she gets and the more isolated she may become. DO NOT change family routines to accommodate the anxiety – you may have to be quite firm with your child about this.

**Most parents would like to reassure their child that she is all right.** Unfortunately, the more you reassure somebody, the more she is likely to come back for further reassurance – so that repeated reassurance actually encourages your child to express (and feel) her anxiety more. So keep reassurance to a minimum – restrict yourself to only ONE reassuring statement; then move on to a distracting activity. After this, refuse to give any more reassurance. Instead you could say, for instance, 'We have already talked about that, and I don't need to say any more'. Use distracting activities at times you notice your child becoming anxious. If a child keeps coming back to anxious thoughts, you can point this out to her: 'It is your worried thoughts making you feel like this'.

**If your child says she needs to share worrying thoughts with you, you can set a specific time each day when she can do this,** for instance for 20 minutes after tea. You can then discuss the events of her day and listen to her anxieties and worries arising from these. It is best NOT to do this at bedtime. If she tries to talk at other times, ask her to wait for the worry-talk time and move away from the subject.

If your child asks for a detailed agenda of what you are doing or where you will be when she is not at home (for instance at school), resist giving her too much detail. This is just a way of increasing the reassurance she can get from you and will only increase her anxiety in the long run. Similarly, do not phone or text your child at regular times to check that she is all right or to tell her that you are all right. This would be another way of giving repeated reassurance.

**As a parent, you need to take every opportunity to point out your child's abilities and enhance her confidence.** However worried you may be about her anxiety, you need to provide a good role model of confidence and help the child to see how the world can feel like a safe place to be in (if you take reasonable precautions). It is a normal part of everyday life for your child to experience some anxiety.

**If a child has a specific worry,** set small goals with a view to increasingly facing up to it. For instance, if a chief source of anxiety is going into town to shop, gradually take an initial step and then increase this activity: initially, you may plan to go to just one shop and then come home; then two shops, and so on. Praise the child for any confident behaviour and any attempts at managing her own anxiety. Such strategies may lead to things appearing worse before they get better – if you persevere, you will begin to see improvements.

**If the main problem is anxiety about going to school,** it is essential to coordinate your efforts with the school staff. For instance, if your child frequently gets sent home from school feeling unwell and then recovers at home, obtain the agreement of school staff to her staying on the school premises despite feeling ill.

**Remember:**
- no repeated reassurance
- use regular worry-talk times if necessary; at other times use distraction
- emphasise your child's abilities whenever possible
- emphasise the safety of the world around us as much as possible
- do not confirm your child's anxiety by showing yours
- do not collude in your child's avoidance
- challenge avoidance in small achievable steps
- praise any success
- work together with other involved adults.

## For parents

- Mental Health Foundation. *The Anxious Child*. London: The Mental Health Foundation; 1997.
  This is a small booklet giving convenient basic information; it is now out of print but free to download from: www.mentalhealth.org.uk/publications/the-anxious-child
- Creswell C, Willetts L. *Overcoming Your Child's Fears and Worries: a self-help guide using cognitive behavioural techniques*. London: Robinson Publishing; 2007.
- Lewis D. *Helping Your Anxious Child*. London: Vermilion; 2002.

## For younger children

- Cooper H. *The Bear Under the Stairs*. London: Picture Corgi; 2008. This monster-in-a-closet is a daytime fear. He lurks in corners and under the table. William feeds him, with eyes shut tight. He tosses offerings under the stairs until the smell alerts his parents and William explains. Then he and his mother clean out the cupboard.
- Prater J. *Tim and the Blanket Thief*. New York, NY: Atheneum; 1993.
  In the middle of the night, shy, unadventurous Tim courageously pursues and does away with the blanket thief. Triumphantly, he returns home not only with his own security blanket, but also the beloved blankets and toys of a number of other children.
- Rosen M, Oxenbury H. *We're Going on a Bear Hunt*. London: Walker Books; 1993.
  All members of the family have to be brave in this story.

## For children and adolescents

- Huebner D, Matthews B. *What to Do When You Worry Too Much: a kid's guide to overcoming anxiety*. Washington DC: Magination Press (American Psychological Association What to Do Guides for Kids); 2005.
- Ironside V, Rogers F. *The Huge Bag of Worries*. London: Hodder Children's Books; 2004.
- Stallard P. *Think Good – Feel Good: a cognitive behaviour therapy workbook for children and young people*. Chichester: WileyBlackwell; 2002.

## For professionals

- Stallard P. *A Clinicians Guide to Think Good, Feel Good: using CBT with children and young people*. Chichester: Wiley-Blackwell; 2005.
- Stallard P. *Anxiety: cognitive behaviour therapy with children and young people*. London: Routledge; 2008.

# CHAPTER 21

# School refusal

## INTRODUCTION

### Definitions

*School refusal* is *a child's avoidance of school which is known to his parents.* It is almost always linked to *anxiety*, although this may only be apparent when attempts are made to get the child back to school. For this reason, it is sometimes called *school phobia*, but this term implies that the anxiety is all related to school, whereas the anxiety may be at least partially home-based (for instance about what might happen at home if the child is not there). Examples of situations giving rise to school-based anxiety include: bullying (*see* Chapter 22), exercise-induced asthma, and undetected specific or general learning difficulties (*see* Chapter 35).[1] Examples of situations giving rise to home-based anxiety include: recent parental separation (the mother has just walked out, so the child fears that father will too); parental illness (the mother has severe recurrent asthma, requiring frequent ventilation); and illness in another family member (a close grandmother has just died unexpectedly of an undiagnosed illness, so the child fears mother will too). In general, such fears (which may in themselves be entirely proportionate to their cause) are expressed by the behaviour rather than in words – which can give rise to difficulties in assessment and management.

In contrast, *truancy* is *the wilful avoidance of school without parental knowledge,* and is far less likely to present to child mental health professionals outside the school (it *is* likely to concern police). Usually, the child leaves home as if to go to school but does not go there, or attends only for registration and then wanders off the premises, usually with others: they often get up to something while evading adult supervision. As an over-simple generalisation, school refusal is associated with disorders of emotion, and truancy with disorders of conduct.[2]

*Hybrid conditions* occur, including elements of both truancy and school refusal. For instance, children in families where there is a negative attitude to school attendance may have particular difficulties: multiple children in the same family may fail to attend, and sometimes multiple families on the same housing estate. Some parents may condone a young person taking days off school without asking the school – in order to go fishing, do a night-time job or just for a family holiday. Wilful avoidance of school may occur with parental acquiescence, for instance if the parents do not want to push the young person too hard for fear of an aggressive reaction. Anxiety-based non-attendance may occur without parental knowledge.

Because the term 'school refusal' presumes almost as much about the child as 'school phobia', and because of the potential overlap between school refusal and truancy, many professionals prefer to use the term *'school attendance difficulties'* or something similar. This however is a broader term and includes children who have what the school would regard as a legitimate reason, such as a chronic illness.

Figure 21.1 shows some of the factors involved in the development of school refusal and truancy, so as to demonstrate the differences and potential overlap between the two.

### Ways of understanding school attendance problems

Both school refusal and truancy can be thought of in terms of their *function*.[3] Contributory factors may include *negative reinforcers* (things to be avoided) such as bullying or teacher criticism or other socially aversive experiences; and *positive reinforcers* (things that make you want to do more of them), such as spending time at home with a parent, spending time at home with a computer, or spending time elsewhere with friends.

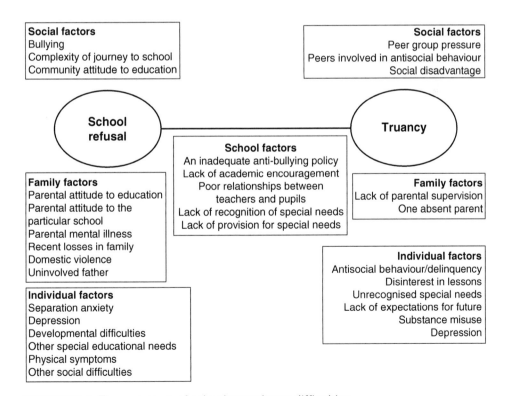

**Social factors**
Bullying
Complexity of journey to school
Community attitude to education

**Social factors**
Peer group pressure
Peers involved in antisocial behaviour
Social disadvantage

School refusal

Truancy

**School factors**
An inadequate anti-bullying policy
Lack of academic encouragement
Poor relationships between
teachers and pupils
Lack of recognition of special needs
Lack of provision for special needs

**Family factors**
Parental attitude to education
Parental attitude to the
particular school
Parental mental illness
Recent losses in family
Domestic violence
Uninvolved father

**Family factors**
Lack of parental supervision
One absent parent

**Individual factors**
Separation anxiety
Depression
Developmental difficulties
Other special educational needs
Physical symptoms
Other social difficulties

**Individual factors**
Antisocial behaviour/delinquency
Disinterest in lessons
Unrecognised special needs
Lack of expectations for future
Substance misuse
Depression

**FIGURE 21.1** The spectrum of school attendance difficulties

It is the authors' experience that many young people find school difficult for a variety of reasons, and sometimes it seems *the only sane thing to do* is refuse to attend school: the anxiety may be thoroughly justified. School refusal may therefore be seen as a reflection of systemic difficulties in gearing educational settings to the needs of *all* pupils, as much as a reflection of individual (or family) mental health problems. Some young people who refuse to go to school or play truant do not appear to have any significant mental health problem.

**BOX 21.1** Case Example

Philippa is 14 years old and beginning year 10 (her first GCSE year) when she stops going to school at all. She had some attendance difficulties in Year 8, but these resolved after some fairly intensive support from her head of year. School staff are concerned that Philippa's mother does not seem keen on getting any professional help with this: she refuses to meet with the educational welfare officer because he made a threat of legal proceedings two years ago.

At the request of Philippa's new head of year, and with her mother's permission, the community school nurse visits her at home to try to understand what is going on. Philippa is initially reluctant to explain her difficulty with school, saying only: 'You're not going to make me go back!' So, with Philippa's permission, the nurse starts by talking with Philippa's mother, alone.

Philippa's father left home when she was nine years old, and initially kept in regular contact, but for the last year there has been no contact, partly because he lives so far away, and partly because Philippa does not like staying with him. Philippa's best friend moved away six months ago, and since then she has had difficulty getting on with others at school. Philippa has not owned up to bullying, and won't let her mother see her Facebook page, but her mother strongly suspects she is being treated badly by peers at school. Philippa also has a long history of personality clashes with about half her teachers, although she currently gets on very well with her English and art teachers. She has always had difficulty understanding mathematics and science.

The community school nurse then has a chat with Philippa, without asking most of the questions she would really like to (listed below in the assessment section). She asks Philippa whether it would be all right to talk with her teachers at school and Philippa shrugs her shoulders: 'I suppose so'. The nurse asks a leading question: 'Your mother says you don't get on with people at school. Is that right?' – to which Philippa also shrugs her shoulders: 'You could say that'.

The community school nurse discusses what she has learnt from Philippa's mother with her teachers, who confirm that Philippa does seem to have become ostracised since her best friend left the school, and that she can be a big problem in some classes (for instance getting into a strop, being rude to the class teacher and walking out), although she gets on well with her English and Art teachers. Philippa was found while in Year 8 to have a specific numeracy difficulty, which may explain her difficulties with maths and science.

The community school nurse seeks advice from the primary mental health worker, then returns to Philippa and her mother, who are both very reluctant to be referred to specialist CAMHS. Philippa refuses to consider a gradual return to school and the community school nurse suspects there is more that she is not being told. Both Philippa and her mother want home tuition, but the nurse advises that the local education authority prefers a local tutorial centre for secondary school pupils for whom ordinary school is too stressful. This requires a referral to the school's educational psychologist, to which Philippa and her mother reluctantly agree. They have to wait a further eight weeks for the educational psychologist to do a home visit, which results in a referral to the tutorial unit.

The head teacher there is reluctant to accept the referral initially, as she says not enough has been tried to get Philippa to return to her proper school. However, the community school nurse is able to persuade the head teacher that nothing will be achieved by postponing things, and Philippa is given a place to start in the following term. She eventually does very well there, and subsequently passes three GCSEs with good grades.

## Involved professionals

It is the role of *educational welfare officers* (alternatively known as educational social workers) to keep under review the attendance of pupils in all the schools to which they are attached. They therefore have an important task in supporting parents of children who are having difficulty attending. Some parents may however find it easier to seek help from *community school nurses*, because of the policy of some educational welfare services to employ threats of court proceedings at an early stage. This may be effective for some families – perhaps for those parents who do not discharge their duty to get a child (or children) to school – but is unlikely to be helpful when there is a significant component of child anxiety or parental mental health problems, which threats of legal action are likely to exacerbate. In some areas, the school educational psychologist may also be involved in helping young people who find school attendance anxiety-provoking. Depending on local referral practices, the *primary mental health worker* or *specialist CAMHS* may accept referrals not only from the child's general practitioner, but also from the educational welfare officer, the educational psychologist, the community school nurse, other staff at the school and in some areas a parent. School refusal is more likely to present to child mental health professionals than truancy – hence the emphasis in this chapter on that end of the spectrum.

## PRESENTATION

School refusal often presents with physical symptoms, such as nausea, recurrent abdominal pain, headaches or diarrhoea. The child's parents may take him to the general practitioner, thinking there is something physically wrong. These symptoms can be seen as an expression of the child's distress at being forced to go to school, and often subside once the child is sure he does not have to go to school that day – or else they will subside on Friday evening! The general practitioner has a very important role in the management of school refusal: assessing the severity of these symptoms; investigating and referring as necessary (but minimally); and, when appropriate, reinforcing the efforts of other professionals and the child's parents to get him back to school.

**BOX 21.2** Case Example

Tracy is a nine-year-old girl who has had difficulty making friends at her new school since her family moved house a year ago. She develops a flu-like illness towards the end of winter, leading her to have several weeks off school feeling ill. Her mother brings her to the general practitioner to find out what is wrong. A diagnosis of a persisting viral illness is made, although a blood test for glandular fever is negative. The general practitioner advises continuing symptomatic treatment and a return to school as soon as Tracy feels able.

The symptoms persist into the Easter term, when Tracy can manage only a random two to three half-days of school per week. Her mother is concerned about a serious underlying illness, while her father is insistent that she should just get back to school. Her general practitioner retakes the history, which reveals that Tracy perks up at weekends, but seems worse on Sunday evenings. He repeats a full examination, does a few more simple tests, and is then able to reassure both parents firmly that there is unlikely to be anything the matter other than the residual viral symptoms. He encourages them both to put more effort into continuing Tracy's gradual return to full-time school.

The parents arrange to meet with school staff and together they agree that Tracy will start from the beginning of a reintroduction programme. She will go into school initially for an hour every day with a view to increasing her time there gradually. A teaching assistant that Tracy likes is identified as a point of contact for her. Tracy can see her each day if she wants to discuss how her day is going or if there are any problems. Her mother drives her in, so that Tracy does not have to cope with the school bus – which emerges as a particular difficulty for her. It also turns out that the social pressures of lunchtime are too much for Tracy, so once she can manage afternoons, her mother visits the school for the lunch break, and they eat in the car or the local park together, depending on the weather. Her father helps her keep a diary of her progress on the family computer.

Tracy makes slow but steady progress over the course of the next several months, from one lesson a day to five half-days and by the end of the summer term is attending full-time. Once she is attending school full time, she is able to experiment with journeys on the school bus and lunchtime with the friends she has by now made.

## Prevalence

Minor forms of school refusal are common, and are likely to involve the general practitioner or community school nurse in assessing anxiety or physical symptoms.

Complete refusal to attend school is rarer, and is likely to involve referral to a primary mental health worker or specialist CAMHS. The prevalence is roughly equal in girls and boys.[4] The condition can occur at any age, but is said to peak at times of school transition (ages five and 11), and at 14–15 (penultimate GCSE years). There may be a history in at least one parent of anxiety or depression.[5]

## ASSESSMENT

### History

What is the pattern of school attendance, associated somatic symptoms, and expressed anxiety, if any? Enquire specifically about the autonomic symptoms of anxiety shown in Box 21.1 of Chapter 20 on Anxiety, Worry, Fears and Phobias. The timing of the symptoms is particularly important: are they worse during the morning, especially on Mondays or Sunday evenings? Are they better later on in the day (especially on Fridays) or at weekends?

Is there a history of *separation anxiety?* Were there difficulties separating at nursery school/primary school/going to stay with friends? What experience has the child had of managing in group social situations? How easy has he generally found it to make new friends or cope with new social groups?

Is the school attendance difficulty long-standing, or has it developed recently? Are there any academic difficulties at school? Does the child have any other difficulties such as an Autistic Spectrum Disorder? What is the current pattern of friendships (social isolation, or close friendships at school and outside school)? A withdrawal from friends or a lessening of interest in previously enjoyed activities may indicate a *depressive disorder* (*see* Chapter 26 on Depression).

A common *family pattern* in school refusal, particularly at primary or middle school, includes a mother who may appear 'overprotective' to professionals, responding with significant anxiety to each of her child's symptoms, and an absent or uninvolved father. In an extreme case, the mother may have agoraphobia, and may need one of the children, often the youngest, to stay at home to help her get out. However, this stereotype needs to be approached with curiosity. What might be making the mother protective? Is her child genuinely more at risk than other children? Does the school have difficulties understanding this child's specific needs? Has the mother herself had experiences of not being adequately protected? Secondary or high school refusal is more likely to be associated with a lack of parental involvement or authority.

A brief individual interview with the child is more likely to elicit *sources of anxiety* and possible *depressive symptoms*, but many of the same questions can be asked in the presence of parents. Bullying at school is possibly the single most important possibility. A direct question such as: 'Is anyone at school calling you names, or doing anything nasty to you?' may be enough to start a conversation, but sometimes the child may be extremely reluctant to betray the bullies for fear of retaliation (*see* Chapter 22 on Bullying). The journey to school can also be highly aversive to some children: severe victimisation can occur on the school bus.

The child's *anxieties* may not be at all clear even to the child himself – apart from the fact he doesn't wish to go to school. Can the child say what he thinks may be scary? What is the hardest thing about going to school? Which parts of the school day are all right? Are there any things about school that he enjoys? Is there a friend or teacher, class or activity he particularly likes? What does he do when he feels anxious or ill at school? What else could be done to help him stay in school and deal with this? Are there things going on at home that worry him? What makes it so hard to leave home in the morning?

There may be clues in the **recent family history** to the child's anxieties about what might happen when he is not at home: have there been deaths or illnesses in the extended family recently? Has either parent been unwell? Is there any evidence of domestic violence?

Try screening questions for **depression**, such as: 'Do you think you're unhappy at the moment?' or 'What do you enjoy doing at the moment?' This can lead on either to a question about a reduction in interest or social activities (and so more questions about depressive symptoms), or to questions about what the child does when *not* at school, which can sometimes reveal unexpected positive reasons for being off school.

## MANAGEMENT

Establish with the parents that *they want their child to return to school.* If they do not, then there is little point in proceeding. For instance, if they think he is too ill, irrespective of your view that he is not, then a paediatric referral may be necessary to give adequate reassurance. If the parents believe that school is doing their child no good, then they may be prompted to act by the statistic that roughly 40 days per year absence leads to a reduction of at least one grade across all GCSEs. If not, they will have to answer to the Educational Welfare Service, who may decide to use court proceedings – unless the parents can either find a more appropriate school, or teach their child at home.[6] For some well-motivated families, regularly inspected home schooling can be a satisfactory way of evading legal action and avoiding the well-meaning interference of professionals. Social contact for the child may be provided by meeting up regularly with other families in a similar situation.

If the parents request **home tuition**, explain that this is unlikely to be in the best interests of the young person: it is likely to increase his social isolation and can exacerbate any tendency to avoid anxiety-producing situations or confront social challenges. It can also make him even less motivated to get back to school. So *home tuition should be used only as a last resort.*

If parents agree they want the child back in school, then it is essential that they not only **collaborate** with each other, but also keep in constant contact with the school. It is important to start getting the child back to school as soon as possible, but also to enable this to happen gradually, so as to accustom the young person to the changes involved, and the likely increase in anxiety these can bring. The longer a child is out of school, the harder it is to get him back. So discourage any post-ponement of the initial return to school, such as for a family holiday or until the beginning of the next term (when it will almost certainly be more difficult for the child to return). If there are any family issues making it difficult for both parents to be involved or to cooperate, these may need some intervention, even if it is only to emphasise how much easier things will be to sort out with two parents pulling in the same direction – but such issues should not be allowed to delay the start of school return. (As suggested in the case example in Box 21.1 and Figure 21.1, an absent parent can make things more difficult, but he or she should nevertheless be involved if at all possible.)

To establish the necessary working relationship with school and agree a time-table for return, a *meeting* should be arranged as swiftly as possible in school, including ideally any involved professionals, the class teacher, both parents and the child. School refusal is one condition for which a delay in intervening really *does* matter: so if there is a long waiting list for specialist CAMHS, it may be better to get on and sort things out, in preference to referring. Many schools have a pas-toral care team experienced in supporting children in their return to school, often including the special educational needs coordinator.

Issues to discuss at such a meeting include the following.

➤ The overall aim should be that the child return to school full-time as soon as he can be helped to do so – which should be agreed between parents and school staff.

➤ Also, deal with any identified sources of anxiety as far as possible: for instance, get the parents to insist the school should put a stop to any bully-ing, ask the school to provide extra help with any specific learning difficul-ties, or ask parents to have a discussion with the child about the deaths and illnesses in the family (they may have been protecting the child from such a discussion, inadvertently encouraging fears of something similar happening to mum or dad).

➤ Get the parents to negotiate with the school the smallest possible first step. This might be merely a trip to the school premises out of school hours without going in, or an hour spent in the special needs room or library.

➤ Encourage the parents to support the child in this. Warn that this, or subse-quent steps, may increase anxiety and either worsen physical symptoms or lead to anger and aggression.

➤ Enable the parents to negotiate with the school and child what the next steps should be: if one proves too big, break it down into smaller components. They must pay attention to practical details, such as what happens in school if a par-ticular step is too much: there must be a face-saving alternative to having to run out of school, such as going to a particular member of school staff.

➤ Praise the parents and child for any small success, and ensure the parents also praise the child effusively.

➤ Be alert for depression – more likely in secondary than primary school children – which may require more specialist input (*see* Chapter 26 on Depression).

➤ Low self-esteem can be more easily dealt with, for instance by extra help in class for any specific learning difficulties and consistent encouragement from parents and teachers.

➤ Predict relapse: once the child is back at school, returning to school after a period off due to sickness or school holidays may lead to a temporary re-emergence of symptoms; if expected, these should be easy to manage promptly using the above strategies.

This sort of simple behavioural package is most likely to be effective if applied early, and is generally more acceptable to children, families and school staff than other types of treatment package.[7]

## REFERRAL

When the problem is mild and not entrenched, many parents can adopt this sort of plan with the minimum of support and guidance. An incipient school attendance problem can be dealt with at an early stage, when this is easiest. Pitfalls include prolonged attention to physical symptoms, which in some cases can allow a pattern of school refusal to become established. Paediatric referral may be necessary at an early stage for parents who won't accept a general practitioner's reassurance.

Some parents may find it difficult to collaborate effectively with each other or with the school. An energetic educational welfare officer or primary mental health worker may be able to broker agreements. If the extent of the child's anxiety or depression is severe and likely to make return to school very difficult, then a primary mental health worker should be consulted or a referral to specialist CAMHS may be necessary.

## PROGNOSIS

The prognosis is better in younger children, and in those who have been out of school for only a short time. Behavioural treatments, of the sort previously described, are effective in most primary school children with a short history. The case example described in Box 21.2 above shows how parents can be very effective if they work together and with the school when prompted by early intervention (in this case by the general practitioner). Tracy could easily have developed fullblown chronic fatigue syndrome (*see* Chapter 29) or an established school refusal problem, but neither of these labels proves necessary, and she is able to return to a normal developmental pathway.

Secondary school children do worse, particularly if they have been out of school for more than a few weeks before any intervention is attempted. After Year Eight or the age of about 14 years, the probability of engineering a successful return to the same mainstream school plummets. Alternative educational placements are often necessary, and are preferable to home tuition (for the reasons mentioned above). These are commonly organised as collections of tutors on one site, so that young people can start off with individual tuition if necessary, but have at least the opportunity for social contact with peers.

Adults who have had school refusal as children seem to catch up in terms of employment with others who have attended school regularly, but have minor psychiatric problems such as depression and anxiety and tend to do less well socially, for instance leaving the parental home later and having children later.[8]

**BOX 21.3** Practice Points for school refusal

Establish whether the parents accept the need to get their child to school: if they don't, explore alternatives to school return.

Work out the best person or agency to take the lead in helping the child and family: if you are already involved, it may be you, as a delay in getting other professionals involved will most likely allow things to get worse.

Empower the parents to link up with school, both to sort out any sources of anxiety at school, and also to negotiate a return to school in small, manageable steps.

Ensure that the parents have enough continuing support to carry the plan through and revise it as necessary.

## RESOURCES

- Berg I, Nursten JP. *Unwillingly to School.* 4th ed. London: Gaskell; 1996. This book describes the epidemiological aspects of school absence and offers practical help to those who are faced with helping children who fail to attend school.
- Royal College of Psychiatrists. Children who do not go to school: factsheet for parents and teachers. London: Royal College of Psychiatrists; 2004. Available at: www.rcpsych.ac.uk/pdf/Sheet9.pdf (accessed 28 March 2011).

## REFERENCES

1 Naylor MW, Staskowski M, Kenney MC, *et al.* Language disorders and learning disabilities in school-refusing adolescents. *J Am Acad Child Adolesc Psychiatry.* 1994; **33**(9): 1331–7.
2 Egger HL, Costello EJ, Angold A. School refusal and psychiatric disorders: a community study. *J Am Acad Child Adolesc Psychiatry.* 2003; **42**(7): 797–807.
3 Kearney CA. Forms and functions of school refusal behavior in youth: an empirical analysis of absenteeism severity. *J Child Psychol Psychiatry.* 2007; **48**(1): 53–61.
4 Berg I. Absence from school and mental health. *Br J Psychiatry.* 1992 Aug; **161**: 154–66.
5 Martin C, Cabrol S, Bouvard MP, *et al.* Anxiety and depressive disorders in fathers and mothers of anxious school-refusing children. *J Am Acad Child Adolesc Psychiatry.* 1999; **38**(7): 916–22.
6 www.education-otherwise.org
7 Gullone E, King NJ. Acceptability of alternative treatments for school refusal: evaluations by students, caregivers, and professionals. *British Journal of Educational Psychology.* 1991 Nov; **61**(Pt 3): 346–54.
8 Berg, 1992, op. cit.

# CHAPTER 22

# Bullying

## INTRODUCTION

### Definition

Bullying is the intentional, unprovoked abuse of power by one child (or more) in order to inflict pain or cause distress to another child on repeated occasions. It can be either or both of physical and psychological. It can take a variety of forms, such as: teasing or name-calling (the commonest), hitting or kicking, stealing money or possessions, telling nasty stories or rumours, making threats to another person, and social ostracism.[1] Recently, cyber-bullying (bullying using electronic forms of contact) has become an increasing problem; this too can take many forms (*see* Table 22.1).

Bullying, although common, must be considered unacceptable. It is unprovoked, repeated, involves an imbalance of power between the children involved and always causes distress to the recipient – unlike playful activities. It is a covert activity hidden from teachers and parents and can be seen as a form of abuse (peer abuse).

### Distinguishing from normal play

Many children are involved in teasing and/or fighting with their peers. Children are able to distinguish rough and tumble play from bullying. In playful fighting or teasing, playful intent is signalled by laughing and smiling, no hurt is inflicted, all parties enjoy it and the participants stay together until it is over. In contrast, children say it is bullying when children 'gang up' on a single child – who is weaker, subjected to this regularly and upset by it. Children see bullying as aggression for no reason, and even non-participant observers find it upsetting.

### Prevalence

Bullying occurs in most schools and all age groups. Questionnaire estimates suggest that roughly one in four primary school children and one in 10 secondary school children are bullied at least once a term; 10% of primary school pupils and 4% of secondary school pupils are bullied at least once a week.[2] Some children are both bullies and victims. Physical bullying is more common among boys (such as theft, threats of violence or actual violence) and psychological bullying among girls (such as name-calling or ostracism).[3]

**TABLE 22.1** Forms of bullying

| Type of bullying | Examples |
|---|---|
| **Physical** | Hitting<br>Pushing<br>Taking or damaging possessions |
| **Verbal** | Name-calling<br>Insulting<br>Repeated teasing<br>Racist, sexist or homophobic remarks |
| **Indirect** | Spreading nasty rumours<br>Excluding someone from a social group, games or joint activities – ostracism |
| **Cyber-bullying** | Text-message bullying<br>Sending photographs or video clips via mobile phone<br>Phone-call bullying (particularly by mobile phone)<br>E-mail bullying<br>Chat-room bullying<br>Bullying through instant messaging<br>Bullying via websites |

*Cyber-bullying* is becoming more prevalent with the increased use of technology.[4] One study found that 22% of 11–16 year olds had experienced this at least once and 6.6% more frequently.[5] Phone call, text messages and e-mail were the most common forms, and it occurred more outside school. As in other forms of bullying, the perpetrators were usually in the same class or year group and many of the victims had not told anyone about it.

Although the majority of bullying probably occurs in school, some happens on the way to school and back, or in the child's neighbourhood; children may also be victims of crime, such as assault or theft. Young people aged 10–15 years are more likely to be victims of crime (not necessarily reported) than older children or adults.[6] Children may be vulnerable when attending organised group activities, playing in informal groups, or getting on the wrong side of gangs.

Children with obvious medical conditions,[7] physical peculiarities, learning disabilities[8] or other special needs may be especially vulnerable to bullying. Having a stammer or red hair may lead to victimisation. Many children with an autistic spectrum disorder are bullied at some time in their school life. Bullying is a source of distress and may be particularly prevalent among children seeing doctors, nurses or child mental health professionals. Victims may present with psychosomatic symptoms (*see* Chapter 41 on Physical Presentations of Emotional Problems),[9,10] school refusal (*see* Chapter 21), anxiety (*see* Chapter 20), or post-traumatic stress disorder (*see* Chapter 37), and both bullies and victims may present with depression (*see* Chapter 26).[11] Parents are often unaware of exactly what is going on, and teachers often deny that it occurs.[12] Bullying is not just distressing for the victim at the time. A victim may find it hard to concentrate, which can affect his school performance; or he may become socially isolated and anxious – which may pre-dispose to relationship problems and depression in adult life. Bullies often show other forms of antisocial behaviour and are more likely to become delinquent as adolescents and have criminal records as adults.

## ASSESSMENT

Children who are the victims of bullying usually suffer in silence, so it is impor-tant always to consider the possibility. Certain signs and symptoms may indicate a child is being bullied, more often indirectly than directly (*see* Table 22.2). It is important to remember that bullying, like other forms of abuse, can present in a wide variety of ways. Occasionally, bullying only comes to light after a young per-son has committed suicide.

**TABLE 22.2** Ways in which bullying may present

| Behavioural | Emotional | Other |
|---|---|---|
| New requests to be driven to school | A fresh fear of walking to or from school | Reports the 'loss' of books, possessions or pocket money |
| School refusal | An increasing unwillingness to go to school | Comes home from school starving (because of the theft of dinner money or packed lunch) |
| A change of route to and from school | Seems distressed or anxious but won't say what is wrong | Unexplained cuts, scratches or bruises |
| Poor school performance | Appears increasingly withdrawn | Appears to be keeping something secret |
| Starts to self-harm | Starts to show symptoms of depression | Reduced appetite or not eating |
| Asks for or steals money (to pay off the bully) | Cries himself to sleep | Recurrent abdominal pain |
| Avoids leaving home alone at evenings and weekends | Develops nightmares | Headaches |

To find out what is happening, ask the child directly, alone or with his parents. Children may not have the same definition of bullying as you, so 'Have you been bullied?' may not be enough. Even if the answer is consistently no, it can be impor-tant to maintain a high degree of suspicion if there are indirect signs. Try begin-ning with more **general and open questions** such as:

'How are you getting on at school?'
'What do you do at break and lunch time?'
'How do you get to school and back?'
'What after-school clubs or youth clubs do you go to?'

'Does anyone ever pick on you or tease you?'
'If so, how often?'

Then lead on to more *specific questions* such as:
'Does anyone call you names?' or 'Is anyone at school horrid to you?'
'Do you get bullied in any other way?'
'What happens?'
'What do you do?'
'Have you told anyone at home or at school what is happening?'
'If not, why not?'

Ask about Internet usage, access to the Internet outside the home and mobile phone usage. This could reveal some form of cyber-bullying (*see* Table 22.1).

**BOX 22.1** Case Example

The diabetic team cannot understand why Geoffrey, aged 15, keeps coming into hospital with episodes of hypoglycaemia (low blood sugar). They involve specialist CAMHS, whose staff are equally puzzled.

Eventually, Geoffrey admits that his 'friends' at school have been teasing him about having HIV, because he gives himself injections. They have repeatedly threatened to beat him up unless he gives them money, which he has been surreptitiously taking from his well-off parents. He has not been able to tell anyone, although this has been going on for about a year.

It appears that Geoffrey has been giving himself too much insulin at times because he does not know how else to respond to this victimisation.

It is important to convey to the child that it *is* all right to talk about bullying and that relevant adults will try to help him keep safe (he probably won't believe you if that has not so far been his experience). Often, a victim has been instructed not to tell anyone, with the threat that something bad will happen to him or a member of his family if he does tell.

**BOX 22.2** Case Example

Lolly is 14 years old when she joins an Internet chat room. She befriends a 17-year-old boy who persuades her to join him in his tent at a campsite not far from her home, where he takes her virginity. They subsequently meet for a second time, and have sex again.

Lolly eventually tells her parents what has happened, who tell the police, who are able to trace the 'boy' from his e-mails: he turns out to be a 34-year-old man, and there is enough evidence to convict him.

## MANAGEMENT

### Dealing with a child who is being bullied

Once a bullying problem is suspected or has been discovered, it must be taken seriously and not dismissed as part of growing up or a passing phase. Bullying – not only within school but also on the way to and from school – can be successfully tackled as a **whole school problem**. It may also be helpful to develop strategies with the child to be more assertive (*see* 'Kidscape' in the Resources section below) or ignore the bullying more effectively, but it is generally thought that the best way to ensure the bullying stops is for the school to deal with it adequately.

Reassure the child that he was right to tell but also inform him and his parents that **the school has to know what is going on** – in order for something to be done about it. Ask the child who he thinks would be the best person at school to tell. For instance, is there anyone with whom he has a particularly good relationship, or anyone who is best placed to deal with such a problem (such as the head of pastoral care, if there is one). It is best if the child is able to tell this trusted adult himself, but usually the child finds this an overwhelming task, in which case someone has to do so (at least initially) on the child's behalf. You may not feel comfortable contacting the school yourself (teachers sometimes resent being told of bullying in their school, but parents have rights that professionals do not have). If you do not yourself tell the school of your suspicions about bullying, then encourage parents to do so on their child's behalf. Advise parents *not* to bully the school or threaten the teachers – their goal should be to develop a cooperative working relationship so that parents, professionals and school staff can work together to help the child.

Advise parents that bullying is common, and usually makes victims feel helpless – so adult help is required to sort it out. **The child needs to feel able to tell** his parents and teachers enough of what is going on so that they can do something. This means that:

➤ he must feel believed by his parents and professional
➤ he must think he is going to be believed by his teachers
➤ he must believe that his teachers will do something effective about the bullying
➤ he must not be further victimised by the bully or bullies because he has told someone in authority.

For a teacher to say 'don't tell tales' or 'bullying does not occur in our school' is of no help to the child at all. Many **parents need** little prompting **to be assertive** about this issue. Some may need detailed guidance. They should start with the class teacher, form tutor, head of year or head of pastoral care; then if necessary go higher, to the head teacher or governors, and possibly even further: options include involving Parent Partnership, a local councillor or even the local Member of Parliament. Parents may need to ask for the school's anti-bullying policy. Providing the school with some of the publications listed below (in Resources) may irritate teachers but nevertheless be appropriate. Parents may need to go on badgering the school until something effective is done. Schools are legally obliged to pay attention to parents' concerns if these are about the welfare of the child. Parents sometimes need to remind senior members of a school that their staff is responsible for providing reasonable parenting of all children throughout the school day; there may however be some debate about who is responsible during journeys to and from school. If bullying occurs on an unsupervised school bus, parents may need to explore alternative means of the child getting to school.

Other forms of **bullying outside school** may require parents to involve a police community service officer, youth worker or club leader, or the parent(s) of any bullying child. Some police services have individual police officers allocated to a particular secondary school (and its feeder primary schools): if so, this person may be a good point of contact for parents to approach. Parents may require professional support to be able to stand up effectively for their child.

**Common sense measures** may also be necessary. Victims can be taught how to deal with specific incidents. For instance, it may be safer to go to school with a friend, to avoid isolated areas of the school, and not to take valuable items into school.

### Preventive approaches

Given the well-proven link between bullying and young people's emotional health and well-being, preventive approaches to reduce bullying and deal with it early before it becomes an established problem should be strongly supported.[13] Research in Scandinavia[14] and the United Kingdom[15] has evaluated what schools can do – not only to decrease the rates of bullying but also to deal with any existing bully/victim problem. These large-scale studies have shown that the more school staff members do to tackle bullying, the more effective they can be. A range of practical advice and guidance is available (*see* the Resources section below).

Awareness of the problem of **cyber-bullying** and the dangers of Internet usage is essential for anyone working with young people.[16] These Internet interactions are extremely real to young people, being an important part of their lives for most of them, although they may seem in the realm of fantasy to some adults. As stated in the Byron Report, various approaches at different levels are required to deal with these issues, including:

➤ the training of those working with children and young people
➤ age-related restrictions and legislation
➤ empowering young people to manage effectively the risks of the Internet for themselves.[17]

**BOX 22.3** Case Example

Shahin is 15 years old when she falls out with the dominant figure in her friendship group. This leads to a lot of negative comments, many of them excruciatingly personal, being posted about her on Facebook. Her parents cannot understand what is making her so distressed – until Shahin's younger sister explains to them what has happened.

Shahin's parents ask her school head of year for advice about how to deal with this. Fortunately, the school has recently developed a cyber-bullying policy, so the school staff is willing and able to deal with the issue. The insulting comments are removed from Facebook and the instigators apologise to Shahin.

Information and advice on cyber-bullying for young people, parents and teachers is available from a variety of sources (*see* Resources), and some practical suggestions are summarised in Table 22.3 below. The danger in writing such suggestions down is that any guidance is likely to become rapidly outdated by the pace of technological change.

**TABLE 22.3** Cyber-bullying: practical advice

**Advice to children**

Be aware of some of the risks of the web, including:
- not knowing *who* is there (it may for instance be an adult pretending to be a child)
- *dubious* content such as extreme violence, discussions about age-inappropriate sexual activity or pornography
- becoming *addicted* (using it so much that you do nothing much else).

Be aware of ways of keeping safe:
- *don't* disclose personal information such as your home address, phone number or passwords
- *don't* give anyone's credit card details
- *block* anyone who is bullying you – do *not* retaliate or reply.

*Think* before you send a message.
Try to treat others online with *respect.*
If there is something worrying happening online – maybe something you are uncomfortable or unsure about – *talk* about it to a parent, trusted adult or helpline such as ChildLine.
If cyber-bullying *does* occur, keep any evidence and speak out if it is happening to someone else.

**Advice to parents**

Try to take a balanced view of the benefits as well as the risks of new technology.
Try to be *aware* of what your child is doing online.
Try to get involved with your child's online activities enough to *understand* them and talk about them.
Ensure that software controls on the type of content your child can access are installed – and that your child is not bypassing these.
Look for changes in your child's behaviour.
Gather evidence if cyber-bullying is suspected.
Remind your child not to retaliate if he is being cyber-bullied.
Report cyber-bullying to the child's school and the service provider.
If you think the situation is serious enough for your child or another to come to harm, then contact the police.

| **Guidance for teachers** | |
| --- | --- |
| **Preventing cyber-bullying** | **Responding to cyber-bullying** |
| Ensure that the management team dealing with cyber-bullying has enough authority to ensure appropriate actions are taken and includes representatives of relevant stakeholders, including teaching staff, technology staff, pastoral care staff, school governors and ideally parents and pupils. | Make appropriate use of existing anti-bullying policies. |
| | Encourage any pupil identified as a target of cyber-bullying to gather as much evidence as possible of what has happened. |
| Review existing anti-bullying policies to ensure they include procedures and sanctions for dealing with cyber-bullying. | Try to remove any offending words or images from the Internet. |
| | Contain the spread of distribution of content which may prolong or exacerbate the bullying. |
| Promote awareness of the benefits and risks of new technology, for instance through staff training, pupil lessons (for instance in Information Technology and Personal and Social Education) and homeschool events. | Advise the target pupil on steps he can take to prevent a recurrence. |
| | Identify the perpetrator(s). |
| | Take steps to change the perpetrator's attitudes and behaviour. |
| Review and monitor the school computer network and inbuilt safeguards. | Apply technology-specific sanctions (where appropriate and feasible) such as limiting Internet or mobile phone use on the school site. |
| Review and update Acceptable Use Policies relating for instance to use of networked terminals, laptops or mobile phones in school. | |
| Stay up to date as technology advances. | |
| Discuss advancing technology and policy development with pupils and parents. | |
| Publicise cyber-bullying prevention activities to the whole school community. | |
| Celebrate any success in countering cyber-bullying. | |

**BOX 22.4** Case Example

Billy, aged 10 years, is brought by his parents to see his general practitioner as an extra case to be fitted in at the end of morning surgery, having not gone to school because of severe stomach pains. These have been a frequent occurrence in recent weeks. Each time his mother has kept him away from school, the pain has disappeared by mid-morning. Billy's father has taken the morning off work in order to accompany the boy and his mother to see their doctor.

On enquiry, the doctor discovers that Billy has recently changed schools. Since then, he has become rather bad-tempered in the evening, as if the tantrums his parents thought he had grown out of have returned. He has also begun bed-wetting again, having not done so since he was eight.

The doctor decides to explore the idea that Billy may have suffered from the change of school, so asks him in his parents' presence whether he is happy in his new school. Billy grunts in reply, and no one else is clear whether this indicates a 'yes' or a 'no'. Billy becomes slightly more talkative when asked about his friends: he tells the doctor that he still has friends near his home, but has made no new friends at his new school. The doctor asks Billy directly whether he has been bullied: Billy denies this. His mother joins in to say that they have suspected this and have already asked Billy about it. The doctor asks Billy whether anyone has been calling him names and this somehow opens up the conversation. Billy haltingly reveals that this has been happening both on the school bus and in the playground – so often that he has found it difficult to ignore and cannot stop himself getting upset. He will not say who does this and what sort of things they say. Billy has not told any teachers.

The general practitioner writes a note for Billy's parents to take to the school, pointing out that there seems to be fairly clear evidence of bullying and insisting that there should be more supervision on the playground and the bus. The doctor arranges to see Billy and his parents again three weeks later.

At follow up, the parents report a number of meetings with Billy's head teacher. Billy has been able to divulge the names of the main culprits. Their discussions have resulted in a plan that helps Billy tell someone as soon as he is concerned about what is happening to him. At school, this is the lunchtime supervisor, playground supervisor or classroom assistant. The situation on the school bus is proving more difficult to deal with, as there are no adults on the bus apart from the driver.

At further follow up four weeks later, Billy seems happier and his bed-wetting, abdominal pain and temper tantrums have all more-or-less disappeared. Billy's father has altered his working timetable so that he is able to drive Billy to school in the morning, and Billy is getting a lift home from a friend of his mother's in the afternoon.

## REFERRAL

Bullying at school or during the journey to and from school should be dealt with by the school. Some parents may be more assertive than others in putting pressure on their child's school to do this. On occasions, it may be necessary to involve the school's educational welfare officer if the bullying is associated with attendance problems or, if the child has somatic symptoms, the community school nurse, general practitioner or school doctor (often a community paediatrician). Depending on local circumstances, the school's educational psychologist, head of pastoral care, social inclusion manager or school counsellor may also be helpful. Most schools have a senior member of staff responsible for the school bullying policy, who is often the head of pastoral care.

Bullying that has no apparent connection with school may require a different approach, perhaps involving the police or the adults in charge of youth activities. Although in general it is probably best to empower parents to ensure that responsible adults put a stop to the bullying, sometimes the child mental health professional may need to make contact herself with the key person in the community who may be able to do something.

**BOX 22.5** Case Example

John, aged 12 years, is assaulted on his way home from a friend's house, just after dark, by a local gang, in an alley with no overlooking windows or surveillance cameras. His arm is twisted behind his back and he is punched in the face hard enough to give him a black eye. He does not recognise any of his assailants, so when his parents appeal to the policewoman attached to his secondary school for help, she says there is not enough evidence for her to do anything.

In desperation, John's parents approach his general practitioner, who involves the primary mental health worker, who has worked with this policewoman before: both have found the other helpful. They therefore discuss John's predicament to brainstorm how he and his parents could be helped.

The outcome is that John gets to meet a local police community service officer, who discusses with John and his parents how he could feel safe after school. Eventually, John agrees to join some after-school clubs, on condition that one of his parents comes to take him home when they have finished work. On Fridays, there are no after-school clubs, so he has to come home on his own after school (as before), but later on one of his parents takes him to a youth club: the police community service officer introduces him to the organiser and youth worker there. John is not keen to restart weekend football clubs, but agrees to go to a karate club on Saturday mornings. John's father agrees to take him to watch the local Premier League football team when they are playing at home at weekends.

John therefore feels more comfortable about going out when he is not at school, providing he is accompanied by an adult, but he still avoids the alley in which he was assaulted.

There is no further information about the gang members who assaulted John, but the police community service officer makes a point of regularly visiting the area where the assault took place – usually just after dusk. He also persuades his superiors to put up a surveillance camera in the alley. John is aware that he can contact him at any time in the future if he has concerns.

Referral to a paediatrician may be needed if there is doubt about the relevance of somatic symptoms. Emotional or behavioural symptoms may need referral to a primary mental health worker. However, the bullying will not stop because a child has been referred or his name is on a waiting list. Measures to reduce the extent and frequency of bullying must be taken as soon as it comes to light – otherwise, the child's hopelessness will be compounded. A general practitioner or mental health worker who is the first professional to hear of a child's plight is therefore in a key position to initiate an effective response.

**BOX 22.6** Practice Points for managing bullying

Always think of bullying when there are:
- school attendance difficulties
- somatic symptoms occurring on school mornings
- general unhappiness, anxiety or social withdrawal.

Assessment needs to be more than just asking: 'Are you being bullied?'
It is the responsibility of the school to sort out any bullying at school or on the way to school.
If the bullying is exclusively outside school, police or youth workers may need to help.
Encourage parents to put pressure on appropriate adults to help their child.
Involve other professionals only if this does not succeed.
Young people need to be taught about how to keep themselves safe online and how to interact with others via the Internet.

## RESOURCES
### Books for children
- Cohen-Posey K. *How to Handle Bullies, Teasers, and Other Meanies: a book that takes the nuisance out of name calling and other nonsense.* London: Rainbow Books; 1995.
- Elliott M. *Wise Guides: Bullying.* London: Hodder Children's Books; 2005.
- Wilson J. *Bad Girls.* London: Corgi Juvenile; 2006.
  This book, for 9–12 year olds, concerns 10-year-old Mandy, who is being tormented by her classmate Kim and her friends.

### Book for parents
- Thomson J. *Bullying: A Parent's Guide.* London: Need2Know; 2005.

### Charities
- *Kidscape:* This organisation, founded in 1985 by child psychologist Michele Elliott, runs intensive one-day sessions that provide young people with the skills and support to prevent bullying, including for instance: assertiveness training, raising self-esteem, and establishing a support network. www.kidscape.org.uk
- *Bully Free Zone:* www.bullyfreezone.co.uk
- *Anti-Bullying Alliance:* www.anti-bullyingalliance.org.uk
- *ChildLine:* www.childline.org.uk
- *Parentline Plus:* This is a website for parents who are concerned about bullying in their child's life, both outside and within school. www.besomeonetotell.org.uk

## Guidance for teachers

- The *TeacherNet* website – available at www.teachernet.gov.uk/wholeschool/behaviour/tack-lingbullying – has guidance on bullying, including cyber-bullying, and is regularly updated. It hosts a resource pack for schools called *Bullying: don't suffer in silence*, which is available at: http://publications.teachernet.gov.uk/default.aspx?PageFunction=productdetails&PageMode=publications&ProductId=DfES+0064+2000& (accessed 28 March 2011).
- Ofsted is the acronym used for the Office for Standards in Education, Children's Services and Skills: www.ofsted.gov.uk (accessed 28 March 2011). On the website is a report based on children's views called *Children on Bullying*, and another based on inspectors' visits to schools and local education authorities called *Bullying: effective action in secondary schools*.
- Sharp S, Smith P. *Tackling Bullying in your School: a practical handbook for teachers*. London: Routledge; 1994. This is a clear, practical book describing a number of approaches and how a school can go about implementing them.

## Internet safety

- The website www.digizen.org is about how to make digital citizenship safe.
- *Stay Safe Online* – This site contains information about Internet safety for young people, teachers and parents and is produced by Child Exploitation and Online Protection (CEOP). The team from this organisation have also developed a user-friendly site for four years old and above; this provides a guide to Internet safety and safe surfing for young people.
- www.ceop.police.uk
- www.thinkuknow.co.uk
- The *UK Council for Child Internet Safety* (UKCCIS) at www.dcsf.gov.uk/ukccis has prepared some helpful information, including the *Click Clever Click Safe* Campaign Materials and the Byron Report.[18] An offspring of this is *Safeguarding Learners* – available at www.nextgenerationlearning.org.uk/safeguarding – which was established by the British Educational Communications and Technology Agency (BECTA), although this was abolished by the incoming government in May 2010.
- Training for young people to be *Cyber Mentors*, who help other young people fend off Internet bullying, is available at: http://cybermentors.org.uk (accessed 28 March 2011).

## REFERENCES

1 Dawkins J. Bullying in schools: doctors' responsibilities. *BMJ*. 1995; **310**(6975): 274–5.
2 Whitney I, Smith PK. A survey of the nature and extent of bullying in junior, middle and secondary schools. *Educational Research*. 1993; **35**(1): 3–25.
3 Layard R, Dunn J. *A Good Childhood: searching for values in a competitive age*. London: The Children's Society and Penguin Books; 2009. p. 45.
4 Smith PK, Mahdavi J, Carvalho M, *et al*. An investigation into cyberbullying, its forms, awareness and impact, and the relationship between age and gender in cyberbullying [research brief number RBX03-06]. London: Department for Further Education and Science; 2006. Available at: www.education.gov.uk/publications/standard/publicationDetail/Page1/RBX03-06
5 Smith PK, Mahdavi J, Carvalho M, *et al*. Cyberbullying: its nature and impact in secondary school pupils. *Journal of Child Psychology and Psychiatry*. 2008; **49**(4): 376–85.
6 Layard, op. cit. p. 46.
7 Pittet I, Berchtold A, Akré C, *et al*. Are adolescents with chronic conditions particularly at risk for bullying? *Arch Dis Child*. 2010; **95**(9): 711–16.

8 Equality and Human Rights Commission (EHRC). How fair is Britain? Equality, human rights and good relations in 2010. London: EHRC; 2010. p. 321. Available at: www.equalityhumanrights.com/key-projects/triennial-review/full-report-and-evidence-downloads (accessed 28 March 2011).

9 Forero R, McLellan L, Rissel C, *et al.* Bullying behaviour and psychological health among school students in New South Wales, Australia: cross-sectional survey. *BMJ.* 1999; **319** (7206): 344–8.

10 Gini G, Pozzoli T. Association between bullying and psychosomatic problems: a meta-analysis. *Pediatrics.* 2009; **123**(3): 1059–65.

11 Kaltiala-Heino, Rimpela M, Marttunen M, *et al.* Bullying, depression, and suicidal ideation in Finnish adolescents: school survey. *BMJ.* 1999; **319**(7206): 348–51.

12 Dawkins J. Bullying in schools: doctors' responsibilities. *BMJ.* 1995; **310**(6975): 274.

13 Arseneault L, Bowes L, Shakoor S. Bullying victimisation in youths and mental health problems: 'much ado about nothing'? *Psychol Med.* 2010; **40**(5): 717–29.

14 Olweus D. *Bullying at School: what we know and what we can do (understanding children's worlds).* Oxford: Wiley-Blackwell; 1993.

15 Sharp S, Smith P. *School Bullying: insights and perspectives.* London: Routledge; 1994.

16 Sourander A, Klomek AB, Ikonen M, *et al.* Psychosocial risk factors associated with cyberbullying among adolescents: a population-based study. *Arch Gen Psychiatry.* 2010; **67**(7): 720–8.

17 Byron T. *Safer Children in a Digital World: report of the Byron review.* London: Department for Children, Schools and Families and Department for Culture, Media and Sport; 2008. Available at: www.dcsf.gov.uk/byronreview (accessed 28 March 2011).

18 Ibid.

# CHAPTER 23

# Enuresis[1]

## INTRODUCTION

Enuresis can be defined as the involuntary passage of urine in the absence of significant physical abnormality. There is some debate about the age at which wetting should be considered abnormal: as with many other symptoms discussed in this book, it is probably better to think of a continuum rather than a categorical distinction between normal and abnormal. And it is the developmental rather than the chronological age that determines when a child should become dry. In general, 24-hour urinary continence is achieved by three to four years, but roughly 10% of five year olds, 5% of ten year olds and 2% of teenagers still wet, with boys more likely to have persisting nocturnal enuresis than girls.

In view of the frequent occurrence of enuresis, some clinicians may be reluctant to offer treatment to children under a certain age (such as seven years or five years). However, recent guidance suggests that children should not be denied treatment simply on the grounds of age.[2]

Enuresis is divided into nocturnal (night-time) or diurnal (daytime or day and night-time) wetting. Much nocturnal enuresis seems to be due to delay in the maturation of the bladder and associated neural pathways,[3] so that the bladder may overflow easily, or something is not quite right in the signalling process between the sensation that the bladder is full and the trigger to wake up (see below under psychoeducation for more details).

Enuresis is also divided into primary enuresis, which is present from birth, and secondary enuresis, which occurs after a significant period (usually arbitrarily defined as six months) of dryness. Children with known physical disabilities may be unable to achieve continence although they will still benefit from assessment, management advice and support.

## AETIOLOGY

### Genetic

A positive family history is the strongest predictor of enuresis: 75% of children who wet will have a first-degree relative who had enuretic problems as a child. The likelihood of wetting is directly related to the closeness of the relationship, with monozygotic twins demonstrating twice the concordance in enuresis of dizygotic twins.

### Physical

➤ *Urinary tract infections* are associated with secondary enuresis and daytime wetting.
➤ Onset of enuresis in the last few days or weeks may indicate some *other systemic illness.*[4]
➤ *Developmental delay*: Many enuretics are thought to have isolated developmental delay in acquiring bladder control at night. These children often have other areas of specific developmental delay, for instance in motor control or speech. There is also a predictable association of enuresis with generalised learning disability.
➤ *Polyuria* (passing a lot of urine: large amounts frequently) may be secondary to diabetes mellitus (functional deficiency of insulin), diabetes insipidus (functional deficiency of antidiuretic hormone) or disorders of the renal tubules (the part of the kidney that concentrates the urine).
➤ *Faecal retention* may cause enuresis as well as soiling, possibly due to pressure on the bladder.
➤ *Small functional bladder capacity* has been particularly associated with diurnal enuresis.
➤ *Structural abnormalities of the urinary tract,* which can at times be quite subtle, can cause enuresis (usually daytime) and often in the form of stress or urgency incontinence.
➤ Minor degrees of *spina bifida,* affecting just the sacral nerves, can be a cause of enuresis, and may at times go undetected.

It might be expected that seizures would cause enuresis, but children with epilepsy are no more likely to suffer from enuresis than those without. Many parents think their child suffers from enuresis because they sleep so deeply, but wetting can occur in any phase of sleep other than rapid-eye-movement sleep.

### Emotional

Bedwetting can occur as a response to acute stress such as birth of a new sibling, divorce or starting a new school. If this is the case, it is more likely to be secondary enuresis, and tends to be self-limiting. Enuresis may also occur as a response to chronic stress such as an unhappy marriage, domestic violence or sexual abuse. In this case, the picture is often less clear and the enuresis may be primary, implying that the chronic stress interferes with the normal developmental process of acquiring dryness. Social factors may also have an impact on enuresis, for instance impoverished conditions, multiple stresses affecting the parents, having to share beds, or difficulties washing bed linen.

### ASSESSMENT

### History

➤ What is the 24-hour pattern of micturition (peeing/weeing)?
➤ What is the weekly pattern? Is it the same every day? If bedwetting occurs, how many nights per week on average?

➤ Is there daytime frequency (over seven times per day), urgency, straining, pain (dysuria) or accidental wetting?
➤ Are there links with circumstances, such as reluctance to use the school toilets? Do daytime symptoms occur only in some situations?
➤ What is the daily pattern of fluid intake? Does the child or a carer restrict fluids?
➤ What is the lifetime history of bowel and bladder control?
➤ Are there any associated physical problems, such as excessive thirst, diabetes mellitus, constipation, faecal incontinence, specific or general developmental delay?
➤ Are there associated emotional or behavioural problems?
➤ Is there a family history of enuresis?
➤ Is there any relationship to life events?
➤ What are the social conditions, especially the sleeping arrangements?
➤ What are the attitudes of the parents and child to the wetting?
➤ What interventions have been tried so far?

### Examination
A physical examination is not necessary if a full clear history is taken, unless there are specific factors that need investigating.

### Investigation
A multi-stick urine test should be carried out to screen for infection and diabetes only if:[5]
➤ bedwetting started in the last few days or weeks
➤ there are daytime symptoms
➤ there are any signs of ill health
➤ there is a history, symptoms or signs suggestive of urinary tract infection
➤ there is a history, symptoms or signs suggestive of diabetes mellitus.

If the history, examination or investigation suggests more significant disease, then the child should be referred to a paediatrician for further investigation. Prominent daytime symptoms should in general be investigated before night-time symptoms if they co-occur: they are more likely to require paediatric involvement.

### Diary
It may be helpful for the young person or carer to keep a record of where, when and how wetting occurs. This could include the child's fluid intake, toileting patterns and any other daytime urinary symptoms. The structure of the diary should be tailored to the child's particular symptoms. If care is taken over the construction of the diary, it can then easily be converted to a reward chart (*see* below).

### MANAGEMENT OF NOCTURNAL ENURESIS
Assuming that treatable physical causes have been excluded, the following treatment programme is helpful for most children.

### Psychoeducation

The family should be told that bedwetting is very common. The child may not know that in a class of 30 seven-year-olds, it is likely that four children will have difficulties with bed-wetting. It is often very reassuring to realise that others are affected. If there is a family history, the fact that the affected individual grew out of the problem may also be reassuring (depending on how old he was). It is important to emphasise that the child cannot help the bedwetting. If carers want a more detailed explanation, discuss the stages between the bladder filling up and the child waking up (or not).[6]

➤ If the bladder has a small capacity or empties before it is full, it may overflow more easily.

➤ If the kidneys produce a large volume of urine overnight, the bladder is more likely to empty before the child wakes.

➤ If the signals from the bladder do not get through to the brain clearly enough to wake the child, then he will sleep through them.

➤ If he tends not to be easily awoken by anything, then he may not wake up even if these signals are getting through.

### Practical advice

Simple practical advice such as using **plastic mattress covers** and nylon sheets that dry more easily may minimise the inconvenience to the family. A regular day-time toileting routine and good **fluid intake** should be encouraged. Evening fluids should not be discouraged but a sensible regime of intake over the day is advised. This may mean encouraging the child to drink regularly through the day and not missing drinks during school times so that he has to compensate by drinking large quantities in the evening.

Many parents find **lifting** the child out of bed to the toilet at a regular time, for instance when parents go to bed, may decrease the frequency of bedwetting. Some children may not fully awaken when this is done, but nevertheless be able to empty their bladders; others may need to be woken as well as lifted. This approach may work in the short-term for both child and carers; but will not make any difference to the course of the bedwetting in the long-term.[7] A young person with bedwetting that has not responded to a variety of treatments may find it helpful to set an alarm clock or mobile phone to wake himself up and go to the toilet: trial and error may be needed to find the best time.

A parental **negative response** to the bedwetting may make the problem worse: it is important that carers do not punish the child for wet nights or make him feel guilty or ashamed. Conversely, if the child is allowed to come into the parents' bed when he wets or is given a great deal of attention, the family may be inadvertently providing positive reinforcement for the behaviour. In general, a calm, matter-of-fact approach is best. The wet bed should be changed with a minimum of fuss and the child encouraged to have a wash or shower in the morning. No comment should be passed after wet nights but dry nights should be rewarded with praise or a reward chart (*see* below).

The decision as to whether *further treatment* is indicated will depend on the developmental age of the child and how much distress is being caused to the family. For instance, some parents may prefer to wait for the child to grow out of the problem rather than try an alarm or medication.

### Reward systems

Reward systems, including charts or tokens or points, have a relatively high rate of success for bedwetting if they are used properly. They are most likely to work for young children who already have some dry nights each week.

It is important that any reward system should be a positive experience. For instance, promising a reward for each dry night would be unlikely to help a child who has very few dry nights each week. Rewards once given should not be withdrawn, and no penalties should be given. Rewards can be given for any relevant behaviour, such as:

➤ drinking enough during the day
➤ going to the toilet to pass urine before sleep
➤ helping to change the sheets the next morning (as long as this is not enforced in a punitive way).

A simple reward chart can be drawn up by a parent, displaying the days of the week. If the child has the targeted behaviour, a star or special sticker is awarded by the parents and stuck on the chart the next morning. It is essential that the parents are enthusiastic about the chart, as their praise and encouragement when a dry night is achieved is as important an incentive for the child as the star or sticker. It is also important that the child has a group of stickers that he actually likes!

The effect of such a chart will be rapid if the child is going to respond, and the motivation of children and parents is highest in the first few weeks. Such programmes should not in general be continued unaltered for more than six weeks at the most. Regular review is essential. If there has been no effect by three weeks, it is worth discussing with parents what might be making it difficult for the child to use the chart. If there is no clear reason for its not working, the chart should be discontinued and other methods considered.

Some parents may prefer to use a reward system without going to the trouble of constructing a chart. For example, instead of stickers, points or tokens can be accumulated, which can then be exchanged for a bigger reward, such as a trip to somewhere exciting. This can work just as well (*see* also Chapter 13 on Behaviour Management).

### Bedwetting alarms

Bedwetting alarms are the next stage of treatment after all of the above have been tried. They are more likely to be effective if the bedwetting occurs at least two nights per week. But they are not appropriate for all families.

These alarms work on the principle that when the child starts to wet, the urine completes an electrical circuit and sounds an alarm that wakes the child. The theory as to why this is effective is that the child is conditioned to associate relaxation of the bladder sphincter (and thereby fullness of the bladder) with waking up. The aims of alarm treatment are to:

➤ learn to recognise the need to pass urine – even while asleep
➤ wake up when the bladder is full
➤ hold on long enough to get to the toilet.

Alarms can be accessed by specialised clinics, often run by community school nurses. The family's general practitioner or the child's community school nurse will know how the family can access their local service.

There are two types of alarm. One is an alarm mat on the bed and the other type is worn on the child's body. The use of these alarms and the progress of the child should be closely monitored with regular reviews.

In addition to fewer wet nights, early signs of success with an alarm can include:

➤ smaller wet patches
➤ waking to the alarm
➤ the alarm going off later and fewer times per night.

Family members need to be very motivated to make an alarm work. If the parents just turn off the alarm and leave the child without changing the bed he has no opportunity to learn and the parents will complain that the alarm isn't working. It is important, when reviewing progress or lack of it, to ask detailed questions about how the alarm is being used. Rewards (combined if necessary with a diary) may need to be combined with the use of an alarm, for instance for:

➤ waking up when the alarm goes off
➤ going to the toilet after the alarm has gone off
➤ returning to bed and resetting the alarm.

Bedwetting alarms are a very safe and effective way of dealing with bedwetting. Parents can be told to stop using the alarm after 14–21 dry nights. Studies have shown that about 80% of children become dry within two to three months, although there can be relapse after finishing treatment. If the child relapses the alarm can be reinstated until the child becomes dry and further relapses are then very unusual.

If a bedwetting alarm does not work despite all this attention to detail, then it may be effective if combined with medication.

### Desmopressin

*Desmopressin* is a synthetic form of antidiuretic hormone that can be prescribed to make the kidneys pass less urine at night. It comes in the form of tablets or nasal drops but is usually offered as a sublingual melt-in-the-mouth preparation. It can be used at night in children over five years for specific situations, such as a sleepover or a school overnight trip. After the age of seven years, longer-term use becomes more acceptable, in which case it is recommended to have a week off medication every three months, partly to preserve efficacy. Doses for the tablets are 200 micrograms in a single dose at bedtime, increasing if necessary to 400 micrograms; doses for the sublingual melts are 120 micrograms, increasing if necessary to 240 micrograms. Exceeding the maximum recommended dose can cause water overload (not enough fluid is removed from the blood by the kidneys) and, linked to this, a low blood sodium – which could potentially cause convulsions. This is probably the only risk, but nevertheless a dangerous one, which could even occur with normal doses if drinking were excessive. So it is important to warn parents not to let the child drink anything from one hour before until eight hours after taking the medication. Desmopressin is normally taken at bedtime, but some children respond better if it is given one to two hours before bedtime.[8]

### Other medications

If night-time wetting is combined with daytime wetting, anticholinergic drugs such as tolterodine or oxybutynin can be used, but these require paediatric referral. A tricyclic antidepressant, imipramine, could still be used for the treatment of bedwetting as a last resort.[9] Because of potential side effects and the danger of overdose, we would not recommend it.

**BOX 23.1** Practice Points for nocturnal enuresis

> Nocturnal enuresis is common.
> Explanations may be necessary to ensure that parents do not blame the child.
> Management options are in the following hierarchy: use a later one only when the earlier ones do not work:
> - simple management advice about toileting and fluid intake
> - a calm, non-punitive approach with rewards for dry nights
> - bedwetting alarms (require motivated families and attention to detail)
> - desmopressin
> - other medication.

### MANAGEMENT OF DAYTIME (DIURNAL) WETTING

Daytime wetting (diurnal enuresis) is more common in girls than boys. If children develop daytime wetting having been dry, it is important to rule out urinary infection and constipation and also to consider the fact that bladder sensation can be reduced by anxiety. If the child is deliberately wetting in various places in the house, this suggests emotional disturbance, which may need further psychological assessment.

Children who have never been dry by day often suffer from bladder instability and/or a small bladder capacity. As a result of this, they pass urine frequently and with great urgency – and unpredictability. Some girls try to control this by applying pressure to their perineum either by holding it or sitting on a foot. Children tend to reduce their fluid intake in order to try to reduce the frequency of trips to the toilet. This can cause dehydration.

Initial treatment can focus on the parent regularly reminding the child to have a drink and go to the toilet regularly, then gradually letting the child take over responsibility for remembering. This is called bladder training. Once the child can recognise the sensation of wanting to pass urine, the interval between reminders can be gradually lengthened. This aims to increase bladder capacity and decrease frequency (a child over five years should be able to hold her urine for 1½ to two hours: roughly from mid-morning break time to lunchtime at school). Parents need to be encouraged to be positive with their children and praise them for all toileting behaviour. Reward charts may help with young children.

When the child goes to the toilet she needs to be reminded to take time to finish passing all available urine. It can help to get her to wait 20 seconds and then try to micturate (pass urine) again (this is called double micturition).

Fluids are very important and should be encouraged throughout the day on a regular basis. Drinks to be avoided include fizzy drinks, tea, coffee and blackcurrant drinks, because they can irritate the bladder.

It is appropriate to discuss the programme with school staff so that visits to the toilet and regular fluids can be encouraged there, as at home.

Children with daytime wetting are more likely to need paediatric assessment than those with nocturnal enuresis alone: so there should be a low threshold for paediatric referral.

**BOX 23.2** Practice Points for daytime (diurnal) enuresis

Diurnal enuresis has a more varied range of causes and presentations than nocturnal enuresis.

It is worth checking for physical causes, which usually means paediatric referral.

A large group of children respond to bladder retraining. This involves regular reminders, gradually spaced out.

Some children may need complex investigations and/or medication.

## REFERRAL

Referral may be necessary for further assessment and treatment if there is no improvement with initial management: for instance to the local enuresis service or paediatric continence service, or to a paediatrician. Identification of important psychosocial factors may indicate referral to a primary mental health worker, paediatric clinical psychologist or specialist CAMHS service.

**BOX 23.3** Case Example

Simon, aged eight years, is brought to the community school nurse by his mother, Trudy. The family is new to the area. Trudy explains to the community school nurse that Simon has recently started wetting the bed at night (again): he is currently wetting three to four nights per week. On enquiry, it emerges that Simon's parents have recently separated, resulting in Trudy becoming a single parent, having to move house and having to find Simon a new primary school and his three-year-old sister a new nursery school.

The community school nurse advises that the wetting will probably stop in a few weeks, as it is probably due to Simon's adjustment to all his life changes and the associated emotional upset – so it may be possible to avoid any specific treatment. She recommends investing in a plastic mattress cover, and emphasises that Trudy should try not to become upset with Simon if she finds that he has wet the bed, but should keep things as neutral and matter-of-fact as possible while changing his wet bedclothes; she should, however, praise any dry nights. They agree a review in two weeks.

Trudy returns with Simon as planned. The washing machine in her new flat is playing up, and she has found all the wet sheets rather difficult to cope with, so at times has not been able to stop herself shouting at Simon. He is still wetting about three nights per week. The community school nurse goes through a detailed plan that includes: how best to manage the wet beds, a fluid intake regime and a reward chart using Simon's favourite Pokémon stickers. They discuss the possible use of an enuresis alarm or medication (desmopressin) but agree to keep these as options for the next appointment if things do not improve.

The community school nurse asks Trudy how she is coping with all the recent life changes and Trudy is able to talk about how difficult she has been finding life in general since the separation and the move. The community school nurse thinks Trudy might be getting depressed; Trudy agrees to see her general practitioner about this, for possible referral to the practice counsellor.

At the next follow-up appointment four weeks later, Trudy and Simon seem happier and calmer. Simon's bedwetting has reduced to about one night per week, in response to the combination of practical measures and the Pokémon stickers. The community school nurse encourages them to continue with the routine and compliments Trudy for praising and rewarding Simon for dry nights and being able to change the sheets calmly. Trudy has had her first appointment with the practice counsellor and is feeling more in control of her life.

At the next follow-up appointment six weeks later, Simon's wetting has ceased. No further follow-up is arranged, but the community school nurse encourages Trudy to contact her directly in the future if there are any further concerns.

## RESOURCE

- The Enuresis Resource and Information Centre: www.eric.org.uk

## REFERENCES

1 We would like to thank Nina Bunce, Specialist Continence School Nurse, Sussex Partnership Trust, for her advice and help with this chapter.
2 National Institute for Health and Clinical Excellence. *Nocturnal enuresis: the management of bedwetting in children and young people* [NICE Clinical Guideline 111]. London: NICE; 2010. Available at: http://guidance.nice.org.uk/CG111/NICEGuidance/pdf/English (accessed 29 March 2011).
3 Lister-Sharp D, O'Meara S, Bradley M, *et al. A Systematic Review of the Effectiveness of Interventions for Managing Childhood Nocturnal Enuresis.* University of York: NHS Centre for Reviews and Dissemination; 1997.
4 National Institute for Health and Clinical Excellence, op. cit.
5 Ibid.
6 Ibid. Section 2.1.4, p. 29.
7 National Institute for Health and Clinical Excellence, op. cit.
8 Ibid.
9 Ibid.

# CHAPTER 24

# Faecal incontinence[1]

## INTRODUCTION

In older textbooks, this sort of problem was muddily defined, and usually treated as mainly psychological. Worse still, some clinics regarded the problem as unworthy of serious attention. We now think that the majority of faecal incontinence difficulties that present to professionals have a strong physiological component, which needs full attention for there to be any success with management.

**BOX 24.1** Case Example

> A seven-year-old boy is referred for help with faecal incontinence to specialist CAMHS, where the referral is screened and deemed unsuitable. The referring general practitioner is advised instead to refer initially to a paediatrician with an interest in constipation, which she does. The paediatrician does a thorough assessment, explains the physiological impact of constipation, recommends a regular toileting routine and prescribes laxatives. Although it takes a year for the dirty underpants to disappear completely, the boy and his mother are relieved not to have to attend CAMHS.

A lot of confusion is generated by different uses of the same words, so definitions are an essential starting point.

### Definitions[2]

*Faecal incontinence* is defined as the passage of stool in an inappropriate place. It can be divided into *organic* and *functional* groups.

*Organic faecal incontinence* results from an organic disease such as neurological damage. Developmental delay or learning difficulties may be associated with delayed attainment of bowel control, meaning that faecal incontinence is prolonged beyond the age of four years: below a developmental age of four years, faecal incontinence is normal.

*Functional faecal incontinence* can be subdivided into **constipation-associated incontinence** and **non-retentive faecal incontinence.**

*Constipation-associated incontinence* (previously often referred to as *soiling*) is *by far the commonest cause* of faecal incontinence. The child becomes constipated for a variety of reasons, and then the impacted faeces block and distend the rectum, impairing anal tone and faecal retention. Stool, which may be of any consistency, leaks around the mass. Parents often fail to realise the child is constipated, as the stool may be runny or normal.

Secondary psychological problems may result from this that have in the past been seen as primary. For instance, the child may be so ashamed of the soiled underwear that he hides them in drawers, at the back of a cupboard or under the bed, where a parent finds them unexpectedly. Parents may become exasperated, and find it impossible not to be angry with the child (and often themselves) for the smell and mess.

*Non-retentive faecal incontinence* (previously referred to as *encopresis*) is not associated with constipation and occurs in children aged four and older. It can be defined as repeated voluntary or involuntary defaecation in inappropriate places. A small number of children with serious emotional problems will intentionally pass formed stools, or smear them, in places chosen to distress parents/carers, for instance on sheets or walls, and may even write insults with fingers covered in faeces. Learning disability can be associated with stool smearing, which may be exploratory or sensory in nature.

*Chronic constipation* means difficulty or delay in passing stool. There are usually less than three stools a week which are large and painful to pass. Constipation is very common in children and occurs in up to 10% of children. Common causes include:

➤ an anal fissure causing pain on defaecation may result in a vicious cycle with the child retaining stools through fear of pain
➤ rectal loading in itself may cause a fissure
➤ fear of the lavatory or of passing a stool – this may result from punitive potty training, or from an unpleasant toilet that is cold, dark or smelly, or from a frightening incident such as slipping into the toilet bowl[3]
➤ a diet low in fibre or fluid
➤ a battle of wills between child and parents, leading to the child refusing to use the lavatory
➤ medical causes in childhood including hypothyroidism, neurological disorders, Hirschsprung's disease, chronic renal failure and anal stenosis; a history of delayed passage of meconium (more than 48 hours after birth) or constipation from the first few days of life is suggestive of organic disease
➤ drugs – for example, methylphenidate (given for ADHD) or oxybutynin (which can be used for daytime urinary frequency).

## ASSESSMENT

It is important to encourage the use of the term *'faecal incontinence'* rather than 'soiling', which could be considered pejorative. '**Soiling**' is also used interchangeably in the literature with '**encopresis**', leading to confusion.

➤ Get a *description of toileting and faecal incontinence behaviour*.
➤ What are the child's words for faeces and lavatory?
➤ Has the child ever been continent?
➤ When and how did the faecal incontinence start?
➤ How often does it occur?
➤ What happens?
➤ What do the stools tend to look like?
➤ Are there associated physical symptoms, such as abdominal pain, anal pain or wetting?
➤ Are there associated emotional or behavioural problems?
➤ What are the parents' attitudes to the child?
➤ What have they done so far to try and manage the situation?

## MANAGEMENT AND REFERRAL

Usually, after taking a detailed history, a full paediatric examination is not indicated. This is partly because a digital rectal examination can be very distressing for the child – who may already be anxious about using the toilet; and partly because feeling the child's tummy does not necessarily give very much information. Giving a user-friendly explanation of the problem is the first component of treatment (also called *psychoeducation*).

Faced with a child who is experiencing faecal incontinence, it is probably safest to assume initially that he is *constipated*. Firstly, you are most likely to be right (estimates vary from 70% to 90%). Secondly, suggesting an organic cause will relieve the parents and child of blame. You should however make it clear at an early stage (if you are not a paediatrician) that paediatric assessment is important to be *sure* of the nature of the problem. If the family is happy with an explanation involving constipation, you can go ahead and explain how this can cause faecal incontinence; if not, you will probably have to refer to a paediatrician first.

*Explain* to the child and parents together, in appropriately child-centred language, how constipation can lead to faecal incontinence – which many parents initially find counter-intuitive. For example, you could start: '*The parts of the food you eat that aren't burnt by the body for energy go through the whole gut to the end bit – the rectum*'. Draw a diagram of the rectum with a large stool inside stretching the walls apart (this does not need to be anatomically exact: the priority is to engage the child and family in understanding a common cyclical process). '*The rectum becomes very full, so pooing becomes very difficult. The muscles are stretched and so do not work. So poo leaks out, but it is often loose or even liquid poo that gets out, rather than the solid stuff, which tends to get stuck in a large hard lump. It is not only the muscles that stop working properly: the nerves that tell the brain your rectum is full of poo also stop working – so you don't know when you need to do a poo. The poo leaks out without you being able to do anything about it. Sometimes, it looks as if you have diarrhoea when actually you are bunged up*'. It may also be helpful to describe the unintended 'pooing' as something that creeps up on the child unawares. A younger child may like to call this by a name that makes clear its alien intent, such as 'sneaky poo', but an older child is more likely to appreciate an explanation of how his body should work and isn't working. Either way, the problem is *externalised* – made to seem as clearly not the fault of child or parent.

Following an explanation along these lines, paediatric referral may be the next step; or involvement of the general practitioner to prescribe laxatives; alternatively, or at the same time, the following **simple interventions** can be very effective, providing the child and family understand the point of what is suggested.

➤ A **toilet-training programme** can help re-establish a normal bowel habit – and get the stuck 'poo' to come out. The basis of this is encouraging the child to sit on the toilet regularly, maximising rewards for achievable goals, and avoiding all punishment. A useful routine is to wait about 10 minutes after each main meal (or at least breakfast and the evening meal, if this is impractical at school), then sit on the toilet for no longer than five minutes at a time. The child should feel safe and comfortable and may need a foot-stool to support his feet, which should be flat and stable to enable him to push properly. Arms should be relaxed and not holding the seat. The parent should remain close by to prevent the child feeling 'banished'. It should be made as much as possible a pleasant experience, with toys, tapes or stories available. Praise and/or rewards should be given for a good toileting routine – just for sitting for five minutes – rather than for staying clean. Any stool passed in the lavatory can be a source of extra praise or rewards, and any accidents should be simply ignored: any punishment will definitely prolong the problem. A chart can be used, with stickers or stars, but is not essential. The difficulty with such charts is to keep the child interested for as long as it takes for rectal tone to return to normal (which is usually months rather than weeks). Back-up incentives may be needed, for instance for keeping up the pattern of sitting for two weeks.

➤ **Diet and fluids** should be assessed and the child should be encouraged to eat a diet with adequate fibre and drink six to eight cups of fluid a day. Regular exercise will also help keep things moving through the gut.

➤ **Liaison with school** may be necessary to ask for support in helping the child to use the toilet at lunchtimes. If the school toilets are an issue, it sometimes helps to use the staff toilet, which often has more privacy (and is usually cleaner and nicer). The child should also have a change of clothes and wet wipes in a pack at school in case of any accidents.

➤ **Relapse**. There are a number of reasons for such a treatment programme to stall. One of the commonest is failure to completely clear the rectum initially or keep it empty. Another is the length of time it takes for the muscles and nerves in the rectum to return to working properly.

➤ **Continued support**. Because full recovery can take so long, the family will need encouragement to continue with treatment and maintain a positive attitude. Regular review appointments may be necessary, which will make it easy to pick up any setbacks and deal with them quickly.

**Referral for medication**. If these simple strategies on their own do not help the child, or constipation is clearly indicated at the initial assessment, the child will need referral to a general practitioner or paediatrician for medication to treat the constipation. The paediatrician may or may not perform investigations to establish the severity of the constipation (such as a transit X-ray study).

Medications often recommended for the treatment of constipation include:
➤ stool softeners – lactulose, Movicol paediatric plain® (macrogol)
➤ stimulants – bisacodyl, senna, sodium picosulphate
➤ bulk-forming laxatives – ispaghula husk, methylcellulose.

Once laxatives are started, it is important to continue both the medication and the behavioural programme for *at least* three months – usually much longer. Laxatives may be required for *several years*.[4] They may initially cause abdominal pain or increased leakage of stool, and many children dislike the taste, so perseverance requires continuing professional support. If treatment is stopped too soon, the hard lump in the child's rectum will build up easily, as the muscles are still lax. A good sign of recovery is when the child starts to regain bowel sensation and can tell when he needs the toilet.

In severe cases, the child's rectum may need emptying with a disimpaction regime recommended by the paediatrician.

*Further referral:* Those few children who deposit or smear stools may require specialist management. Often such children have other indicators of emotional disturbance, and may be known to social services. Even with this group, however, it is wisest to seek the opinion of a community paediatrician about possible constipation and/or developmental problems before referral to specialist CAMHS.

**BOX 24.2** Practice Points on faecal incontinence

Faecal incontinence can cause considerable distress to child and parents: be sympathetic and attentive to the problem.
The majority of children presenting with faecal incontinence have chronic constipation. This needs appropriate treatment, which may include medication.
A behavioural programme of regular toileting is essential.
Pay attention to diet, fluid intake and exercise.
Recovery can take many months.
Regular follow-up is needed.

**BOX 24.3** Case Example

Joe is seven years old when his class teacher becomes concerned about Joe appearing unhappy in class and on the playground. She notices when he changes for swimming that his underwear is smeared with faeces. Joe has never mentioned to any of the school staff having an accident with his poo. The class teacher speaks to his mother Angela, who is aware of the problem, but has no idea what to do about it. Angela agrees to meet with the community school nurse to discuss what can be done.

The community school nurse makes an initial assessment that suggests Joe is probably constipated. She asks Joe about his poos. He is reluctant to say much, but reveals that the toilets at school are dark and smelly, so much so that he refuses to sit on them. He also confesses that he is being teased a lot, mainly about being smelly.

The community school nurse arranges for the general practitioner to see Joe and prescribe a laxative: he starts on lactulose 10 mL twice daily. She agrees with Angela a daily toileting programme for Joe. He will not sit on the pupil toilet at school, but Angela can make things pleasant for him at home by playing him a story tape and providing a foot-stool to support his feet. Angela agrees to encourage Joe to sit on the toilet for up to five minutes after breakfast and after the family's evening meal. Angela also agrees to ensure that Joe drinks six to eight cups of fluid a day. She thinks it will be more difficult to get Joe to eat a high-fibre diet (vegetables are already a battleground), but agrees to buy only brown bread for the family from now on and encourage Joe to eat more apples, which he likes.

The community school nurse then negotiates an arrangement for Joe to use the staff toilet after his lunch break. She recruits one of the teaching assistants to help Joe sit on the toilet at school for up to five minutes and praise him for staying there. Angela supplies the school with a change of clothes and a packet of wet-wipes in case Joe has any accidents at school. Joe's class teacher agrees to encourage Joe to drink regularly throughout the day.

The community school nurse meets with Angela and Joe initially every two weeks to review progress. The toileting regime works fairly well, both at home and at school, despite some initial resistance from Joe. He needs to be given lots of encouragement. At home, there are still stained pants in the laundry basket. She discovers Angela has stopped giving Joe the lactulose since the first prescription ran out! Angela sets up a repeat prescription.

After two months, Joe announces that he is bored with the regular sitting on the toilet, which is therefore reduced to once daily, just after breakfast. The stained pants have become less frequent. The lactulose is continued. The appointments are reduced in frequency to monthly.

Joe has a setback when his younger sister has to be admitted to hospital, so that Joe has to stay with his grandmother for a week. He recovers from this quickly.

After four months, Joe is doing a regular, well-formed, fair-sized poo every morning. The lactulose is stopped. A review meeting is arranged for two months.

After six months, Joe's mother and teacher report no further problems, and Joe himself seems a lot happier in school. He has joined some after-school clubs and has started to see more friends after school.

## REFERENCES

1 The authors would like to thank Nina Bunce, Specialist Paediatric Continence Nurse, Sussex Partnership Trust, and Professor David Candy, Consultant Paediatric Gastro-enterologist, Royal West Sussex Trust (both at Chichester), for their considerable input to this chapter.

2 Benninga M, Candy DC, Catto-Smith AG, *et al.* The Paris Child Constipation Terminology (PACCT) Group. *J Ped Gastroenterol Nutri.* 2005; **40**: 273–5.
3 W. H. Auden expressed this succinctly in one of his shorter poems:
Avatory, avatory, avatory
The baby fell down the lavatory.'
4 Bardisa-Ezcurra L, Ullman R, Gordon J. Diagnosis and management of idiopathic childhood constipation: summary of NICE guidance. *BMJ.* 2010 June 1; **340**: 1240–2.

# CHAPTER 25

# Tics and Tourette's syndrome

## INTRODUCTION

### Definitions

A *tic* is a sudden, purposeless, repetitive stereotyped movement or *phonic production* – which means a noise coming from the mouth, throat or nose that is not necessarily meaningful. The combination of multiple motor tics with one or more phonic tics is called **Gilles de la Tourette's syndrome**, shortened to **Tourette's syndrome** or **Tourette's**. Combinations of tics that do not quite add up to Tourette's syndrome, or that have not lasted for the arbitrary period of one year, can be called a **tic disorder**. Table 25.1, derived from the Yale Global Tic Severity Scale, gives examples of commonly occurring tics and some of the words used to describe them.[1] Swear words occur in only 10–20% of children and young people with Tourette's, but when they do, are accompanied by distress or embarrassment for the child who utters them, unlike the kind of swearing common in the school playground.

### Comorbidity

Tourette's syndrome is commonly associated (co-occurs) with other conditions such as: obsessive-compulsive disorder; ADHD; autistic spectrum disorder, learning disability and oppositional defiant disorder.[2] Overlapping symptoms may at times cause confusion. For instance, on the borderline between Tourette's and obsessive-compulsive disorder are complex repeated behaviours such as: touching (sometimes repeated for a certain number of times), licking, shouting out in class, pirouetting or smelling.

### Voluntary or involuntary?

Watchers or listeners may attribute intended or implied meaning to the tics (perhaps an intention to annoy or a sign of disapproval), but they are generally meaningless. Another potential source of confusion is the rather fruitless argument as to whether the movements are voluntary or involuntary. Although they may best be regarded as involuntary in order to remove blame, this is probably over-simplistic. For instance, a newly learnt voluntary movement can become a tic; and tics can often be suppressed in novel or demanding environments, only to erupt in more

**TABLE 25.1** Some types of tic (not an exhaustive list)

| Motor tics | Simple (rapid, darting, meaningless) | Complex (slower and apparently purposeful) |
|---|---|---|
| | Eye blinking | Eye gestures or movements |
| | Eye movements | Mouth movements |
| | Nose movements | Facial movements or expressions |
| | Mouth movements | Head gestures or movements |
| | Facial grimace | Shoulder gestures |
| | Head jerks or movements | Arm or hand gestures |
| | Shoulder shrugs | Writhing tics |
| | Arm movements | Dystonic postures |
| | Hand movements | Bending or gyrating |
| | Abdominal tensing | Rotating |
| | Leg, foot or toe movements | Leg, foot or toe movements |
| | | Tic-related compulsive behaviours |
| | | Copropraxia (obscene gestures) |
| | | Self-abusive behaviour |
| | | Paroxysms of tics |
| | | Disinhibited behaviour |
| | | Orchestrated patterns or sequences of motor tics |

| Phonic tics | Simple (fast, meaningless sounds) | Complex (words, phrases, statements) |
|---|---|---|
| | Coughing | Syllables |
| | Throat clearing | Words |
| | Sniffing | Coprolalia (obscene words) |
| | Grunting | Echolalia (repeating what someone else has said) |
| | Whistling | Palilalia (repeating or echoing one's own spoken words) |
| | Animal or bird noises | Blocking (not being able to continue a sentence) |
| | | Disinhibited speech |
| | | Atypical speech |
| | | Orchestrated patterns or sequences of phonic tics |

relaxed circumstances. Many children with a tic disorder or mild Tourette's are able to suppress most of their tics for a period of time, for example while at school, but then are unable to suppress them any longer and have to endure a resurgence of the tics – usually when at home. It seems that tics can for a time be suppressed at will, but the longer they are suppressed, the more irresistible their return. It may be best to regard tics as *mainly* involuntary but *partly* voluntary – giving in to a premonitory urge.

### Causation

Tics used to be thought of as a manifestation of anxiety. It is true that anxiety or tension may worsen tics, as may excitement or illness, but sometimes the need to maintain focus can instead serve to suppress them. There is often a family history of tics, and there seems to be a strong biological basis. A recent theory is that the symptoms of the Tourette's disorder are a consequence of aberrant neural oscillations.[3] By definition, tics are not due to some other neurological disorder such as encephalitis.

### Presentation

The mean age of onset of Tourette's syndrome is seven years (with an age range of 2–21), usually with motor tics such as blinking. Tics are commoner in boys than girls. The tics characteristically wax and wane in frequency and severity over hours, days, weeks, months and years, with no obvious pattern, but are most likely to be severe around the age of 10–12 years. Tourette's syndrome starts to improve in late adolescence or early adulthood, and in general continues to improve with age, although a few individuals continue to experience severe tics throughout their adult life.

**BOX 25.1** Characteristics of tics

---

They may be motor (movements) or phonic (sounds)

They may be simple (rapid and meaningless) or complex (slower and meaningful or apparently purposeful)

They can be voluntarily suppressed for a while

After suppression, they rebound – it may feel as if they have to be *let out*

There may be premonitory sensations: older children can identify a feeling that comes before the tic

They generally reduce during sleep

They may be exacerbated by stress, anxiety, excitement or physical illness

They vary in type: old ones may fade while new ones emerge

They vary in severity: some may be very noisy or intrusive, while others may be very quiet and hardly noticeable

They vary in frequency

---

### Prevalence

Tourette's syndrome used to be thought of as very rare. Recent community studies have suggested otherwise: in one survey, secondary school pupils had a rate of 3% for the Tourette's disorder,[4] and 18% for tics.[5] A more general estimate has been made of 1%.[6] The diagnosis may be missed if it is not considered. The prevalence is even higher in pupils with special needs, especially those with emotional and behavioural disorders or learning disability, presumably because such children are likely to have several of the other conditions listed above that tend to co-occur with tics.[7] Comorbidity (co-occurrence of these other conditions with Tourette's syndrome worldwide) has been estimated as 88%.[8]

**BOX 25.2** Case Example

Roger, aged nine years, is brought to see his general practitioner by his mother, Tracey, who says his teacher has been complaining of his making noises in class. These are mainly sniffing, coughing and throat-clearing. Roger says he has not had a cold, and never coughs up any sputum. There is no history of asthma or nocturnal cough. The general practitioner examines Roger's chest and ear, nose and throat system, which are unremarkable. He suddenly remembers having read an article about Tourette's syndrome, and asks whether Roger has any tics or twitches. Roger and his mother look blank. The general practitioner imitates an eye blink and a shoulder twitch – generating some giggling. Tracey explains that Roger used to blink his eyes a lot, but is not doing it so much now. On further enquiry, it seems that Roger also turns his head to one side on occasions, and feels compelled to touch the side of his desk at school exactly seven times each lesson. The general practitioner asks Roger whether he has ever been bullied or teased, and Roger says he has been called 'weirdo' once or twice, but he has ignored it, and so it stopped. He also asks Roger whether he has any other rituals (like the repeated touching), and both he and his mother say no. The general practitioner explains that he thinks Roger probably has a mild form of Tourette's syndrome, and asks whether Tracey would like a referral. Tracey says she does not want to visit a child psychiatrist, and also that she is not at all keen on medication for it. She agrees that the doctor can telephone Roger's class teacher to explain that the noises in class are probably due to a medical condition, and are likely to be difficult for Roger to control.

Roger comes to the health centre six months later about something else. His tics are about the same, although they fluctuate a lot, but he is no longer getting into trouble with his teacher, who has rapidly dealt with a recurrence of teasing.

## Assessment

Children with tics are often regarded as 'nervous' or labelled as being badly behaved. Bad behaviour is linked to Tourette's, as mentioned above, although it is difficult to explain the nature of this link. Any emotional or behavioural disturbance should not be allowed to obscure the tics: if Roger in Box 25.2 had disruptive behaviour in class, would his teacher be so sympathetic to his repeated sniffing, coughing and throat-clearing? It is important that both tics and Tourette's syndrome are recognised, because of their involuntary component, and the potential risk of teasing or bullying. Although many children need no specific treatment, naming the condition can help the child, parents and others deal with the consequences more effectively – particularly by removing blame.

It is unlikely that a short meeting will reveal much direct evidence of tics. It is easy for you to blink and miss the one tic noticed by the parent – and for both of you to miss or misinterpret the others. It is arguable that tics not noticed by anyone do not matter, but often the child is blamed in class for making some sort of noise, without anyone thinking that this may be a tic. Children often do not notice their own tics, so a careful history is essential. Parents may not know what you mean by tics, so you should demonstrate (which may break the ice, as in the case example in Box 25.2) and perhaps show a list of possible tics, such as in Table 25.1. Find out what word the family have for the tics (habits, twitches, jerks, noises, anxiety . . .).

The history can be supplemented by diary-keeping, but this can become quite a chore for parent and child. Table 25.1 gives a list of the sort of tics to look out for. Teachers' accounts can be helpful, but tics occur less often in the classroom, and teachers may not in any case notice them – or realise they are tics. It is more important to ask about any effects of the tics in school – particularly teasing by other pupils, or getting into trouble with the class teacher (for making noises that disturb the class, or for other repetitious behaviours). If obsessions or compulsions occur, it is worth getting details. Tics may appear to be compulsions, and obsessive compulsive disorder or autistic spectrum disorder may coexist with Tourette's syndrome. The teacher may often interpret a repeated interruption in class as a sign of wilful naughtiness or evidence of obsessionality when it is in fact a tic.

No investigations are necessary, as the diagnosis is made only on the history, so referral is not needed for further tests, but may be needed for diagnosis.

## MANAGEMENT

### Psychoeducation

You may not feel able (or permitted) to make the diagnosis yourself, but suggesting the possibility to parents could help the family see the child's behaviour in a new light, with the help of additional information from the Internet. This may be all the management that is necessary, although many parents will appreciate a definitive diagnosis from a specialist, in which case referral is warranted. It may help to emphasise to parents the difficulty the child has in controlling the involuntary movements and noises, and suggest they discuss this with the child's teachers. If no one has thought of the possibility of a tic disorder, the child may be regarded as merely anxious or simply badly behaved. The child's self-esteem may have taken a battering for some time due to being teased or thought of as 'naughty'. The diagnosis may help others to see the child in a more positive light, and may help the child see himself as neither mad nor bad.

### Individual treatment

A recently developed treatment package titled 'Comprehensive Behavioural Intervention for Tics' has proved effective: a key component is *habit reversal training*.[9] The child is taught to be aware of the urge to tic and to use a competing response; for vocal tics, for example, the child might focus on diaphragmatic breathing until the urge to vocalize subsides. This enables a child to manage the urge to tic so he doesn't have to do it as often or intensely – empowering the child and family to feel more able to cope with the tics. It often makes a big difference to enlist the help of family members. Other potentially effective psychological treatments include:

addressing situations that sustain or worsen tics, relaxation exercises, problem-solving, stress management, *massed practice* (doing a tic so many times that the urge to repeat it is exhausted) and guided imagery. Some young people may benefit from exposure and response prevention for obsessions or compulsions (*see* Chapter 39 on obsessive-compulsive disorder). Some combination of these may be offered by psychologists (or other professionals with relevant training) working in Tier 2 or Tier 3. For a vocal tic, you could try suggesting breathing with the tummy; or, for a motor tic, if the child can identify the urge to do a particular movement, he should try an alternative incompatible movement. For instance, if the tic is a forward head nod, when he feels the urge to do this, he should try to lift his head upwards instead.

### Liaison with school

It is essential that teachers are made aware of the diagnosis, or even the suggested diagnosis, providing of course that parents agree. It is common for tics to occur in the classroom without being recognised as such. Although some children can effectively suppress their tics for the whole school day, many cannot: the resultant teasing or disturbance to the class can benefit immensely from the teacher considering tics as a possibility. An intervention that can help in school when tics cannot be suppressed all day is allocating the child a safe place to tic, with a time-out card that he can show when he feels the need, so as to be allowed to leave the classroom.

### Medication

Medication is probably best left to interested child psychiatrists or paediatricians.

### REFERRAL

It is curious that, by tradition, children with suspected Tourette's syndrome are often referred to child psychiatrists rather than paediatricians, whereas adults are referred to neurologists. This may be because of the high frequency of comorbid mental health problems, or the common use of antipsychotics, which are covered in more detail in psychiatric than paediatric training. However, what is needed initially is a medical diagnosis, which can be provided effectively and rapidly by any doctor. Specialist psychological input may require referral to the local Tier 2 or Tier 3 CAMHS. There seems little value in referring to a team in which no one has an interest in tic disorders, since in our experience this results in under-diagnosis and unnecessary distress for children and parents.

**BOX 25.3** Practice Points about tics

*Tics are common, particularly affecting children at special schools.*
Tics may often be unnoticed or interpreted as something else, meaning that a tic disorder or Tourette's syndrome may go undiagnosed.
The diagnosis of Tourette's syndrome is made by thinking of the possibility and asking the right questions. Occasionally, tics will be observed.
Making the diagnosis of a tic disorder will be enough help for most children and their carers.

Medication is seldom required, but may be necessary if the tics are very noisy or causing significant social difficulties – particularly if these are at school.

Refer to a specialist doctor if there is doubt about the diagnosis, or a clear need for medication.

Refer to a psychologist if the child or carers want behavioural management.

## RESOURCES
### Website
- **Tourette's Action (UK)** – This not only provides children's parties and adolescent camps, but also has resources for professionals such as PowerPoint presentations that can be shown to schools. www.tourettes-action.org.uk

### Leaflets
- Great Ormond Street Hospital has produced leaflets on Tourette's for families and for young people:
  www.ich.ucl.ac.uk/factsheets/families/F010394/tourettes.pdf
  www.ich.ucl.ac.uk/factsheets/children/index.html

### Children's book
- Buehrens A, Buehrens C. *Adam and the Magic Marble*. Pasadena, California: Hope Press; 1991. A fictional story for children about how three boys with disabilities, taunted by peers, find the magical power to cure their disorders.

### Books for parents
- Robertson MM, Baron-Cohen S. *Tourette Syndrome: the facts*. Oxford: Oxford University Press; 1998.
- Chowdhury U, Robertson MM, Whallett L. *Why Do You Do That?: a book about Tourette syndrome for children and young people*. London: Jessica Kingsley; 2006.
- Chowdhury U. *Tics and Tourette Syndrome: a handbook for parents and professionals*. London: Jessica Kingsley; 2004.

### Video clip
- 'I have Tourette's but Tourette's doesn't have me':
  www.tsa-usa.org/news/HBO_Release_apr06_update.htm

## REFERENCES
1  Leckman JF, Riddle MA, Hardin MT, *et al*. The Yale Global Tic Severity Scale: initial testing of a clinician-rated scale of tic severity. *J Am Acad Child Adolesc Psychiatry*. 1989; **28**(4): 566–73.
2  Robertson MM. Tourette syndrome, associated conditions and the complexities of treatment. *Brain*. 2000; **123** (Pt 3): 425–62.
3  Leckman JF, Vaccarino FM, Kalanithi PSA, *et al*. Tourette syndrome: a relentless drumbeat – driven by misguided brain oscillations. *Journal of Child Psychology & Psychiatry & Allied Disciplines*. 2006; **47**(6): 537–50.

4 Stern JS, Burza S, Robertson MM. Gilles de la Tourette's syndrome and its impact in the UK. *Postgrad Med J.* 2005; **81**: 12–19.

5 Mason A, Banerjee S, Eapen V, *et al.* The prevalence of Tourette syndrome in a mainstream school population. *Dev Med Child Neurol.* 1998; **40**(5): 292–6.

6 Stern, op. cit.

7 Eapen V, Robertson MM, Zeitlin H, *et al.* Gilles de la Tourette's syndrome in special education schools: a United Kingdom study. *J Neurol.* 1997; **244**(6): 378–82.

8 Stern, op. cit

9 Piacentini J, Woods DW, Scahill L, *et al.* Behavior therapy for children with Tourette disorder: a randomized controlled trial. *JAMA.* 2010; **303**(19): 1929–37.

# PART 5

# Adolescence

# CHAPTER 26

# Depression

## INTRODUCTION

The term *depression* can be used to refer to a **mood, symptom** or **disorder**. Low *moods* are common, understandable reactions to unhappy experiences. Depressive *symptoms* (such as sad mood, tearfulness, loss of interest or social withdrawal) are also common in children with unhappy life experiences, but may be part of a *disorder*. This seldom occurs under the age of six years, is uncommon in prepubertal children, but increases dramatically with puberty, becoming commoner in girls than boys. Depressive disorder, together with deliberate self-harm and eating disorders, is one of the main reasons for the higher rate of adolescent mental health problems in girls than boys. Worldwide, depressive disorder affects 1–6% of adolescents.[1] *Bipolar disorder* is less common than this, but there is continuing debate about when it is appropriate to make the diagnosis in young people – in other words, how to adapt the adult definition appropriately (*see* below).

The importance of adolescent depression is that:

➤ it impairs functioning (for instance in educational attainment and peer relationships)
➤ it increases the risk of suicide
➤ although it often gets better without treatment, it tends to recur in at least half of cases
➤ having even *some* of the symptoms of depression may be significant in terms of the likelihood of developing a full-blown depressive episode later
➤ it is generally under-recognised.[2]

The last point may be even more of an issue in boys than girls, since depression may masquerade as bad behaviour, irritability or substance misuse, concealing the underlying sadness and hopelessness. Adolescent depression is particularly likely to occur in a young person with a parent who has had unipolar depression or bipolar disorder.

### The depressive syndrome

The syndrome of depression is a pervasive mood disorder, associated with significant suffering or impairment of functioning. In adolescents, the presentation is usually atypical (meaning that it is different from how adults present). For instance, there may be *hyper-somnolence* (feeling sleepy throughout the day and night) rather than difficulty sleeping: adolescents have an increased sleep requirement in any case, associated with the growth spurt. Early morning wakening is uncommon, and initial insomnia can occur with or without depression, but *middle insomnia* is characteristic: waking several times during the night with difficulty getting back to sleep.

**BOX 26.1** Case Example

> A 16-year-old girl presents to specialist CAMHS with excessive daytime sleepiness. She appears to be sleeping adequately at night, and does not seem to have other features of depression, although she is not getting to school for more than half a day at a time, and is hardly seeing any friends – both apparently because of her need to sleep. The recently appointed child psychiatrist is puzzled by this presentation, so refers her to a neurologist for further assessment.
>
> The neurologist suggests she is depressed, and she subsequently responds to a trial of fluoxetine.

Parents and professionals are often fooled by superficial jolliness, or bouts of low mood (rather than continuous low mood), so may find it difficult to distinguish a mood disorder from ordinary moodiness. Irritability may be attributed by parents to hormones or 'attitude' or oppositional behaviour rather than a disturbance of mood. A young person will often conceal from her parents not only how low she feels but also her thoughts about wanting to die.

**BOX 26.2** Case Example

> Rohini is 14 years old when she gradually becomes more irritable with her parents, stops getting top grades at school, and falls out with both her best friends. Her general practitioner refers her to specialist CAMHS without a suggested diagnosis, and the referral is triaged to the primary mental health worker.
>
> Initial assessment reveals marked irritability and some sleep disturbance. Rohini appears to be in a good mood for most of the interview, even when seen on her own. She says she is happy some of the time and unhappy some of the time; and denies any suicidal thoughts. She is offered some individual therapy, which she agrees to take up, although it cannot begin immediately.
>
> Before the date for Rohini's first individual session has arrived, she is admitted to the paediatric ward following an overdose of 15 paracetomol tablets. During the assessment the morning after, she admits to very low moods and associated frequent suicidal thoughts during the last three months: she did not admit this in the first interview, as she thought her parents would be told, and she did not want to worry them. She admits to being very good at pretending to be jolly, even when she feels quite desperate inside.

Adolescent depression may present predominantly as *anxiety*, which overlaps with depression in 30–75% of cases (*see* Chapter 20 on Anxiety, Worry, Fears and Phobias).[3] *Bodily complaints* are also common, including not only tiredness/low energy, but also musculoskeletal pains[4] and headaches (mainly in girls)[5] (*see* Chapter 41 on Physical Presentations of Emotional Distress).

**BOX 26.3** Case Example

Imogen is 15 years old when her headaches start to severely disrupt her GCSE work. Her general practitioner refers her to a paediatrician, who thinks the headaches are more likely to be stress-related rather than migraines. Under pressure from Imogen's well-read parents, the paediatrician performs an MRI scan of Imogen's brain, which is normal. They continue to pressurise her to *do something* about the headaches, so she asks her child psychiatry consultant colleague for advice. The child psychiatrist, who has worked with the paediatrician for some years, initially suggests some anxiety management techniques, but the paediatrician says she is unlikely to persuade either Imogen or her parents that these will help. The child psychiatrist says she has seen stress-related headaches respond to fluoxetine even when there are no other apparent symptoms of depression or anxiety. Given that Imogen's parents are very reluctant to see a mental health professional, he suggests the paediatrician should prescribe a trial of fluoxetine 20 mg daily.

The trial is surprisingly successful, and Imogen gets good grades in her GCSEs without interruption from headaches. Her parents are keen for her to come off the medication as soon as possible, but the child psychiatrist (via the paediatrician) persuades them to wait until the summer holidays after Imogen's AS levels. She is able to withdraw the fluoxetine then without any recurrence of her headaches.

The presentation of depression varies with the age of the child. In under-11s, the picture may be different even from adolescents. Sadness and helplessness can be prominent presenting features of depressive disorder in six to eight year olds. Depressed children between the ages of eight and 11 years tend to describe feeling unloved and unfairly treated (which may or may not be true from the perspectives of adults). Running away from home is more likely as an expression of low mood than self-harm in under-11s and could be seen as a self-harm equivalent (but the professional needs to consider whether there may be a good reason for the child to run away, such as domestic violence or other forms of abuse). If self-harm does occur, under-11s are more likely to think of jumping out of a window or running in front of a car; over 11 years, overdoses and cutting become much more common; self-hanging may occur from nine years onwards. The younger the child, the less the chance of completed suicide. Presenting symptoms of depressive disorder after the age of 11 years are more likely to include guilt and despair. Table 26.1 summarises the symptoms to look for. Depression can be categorized into mild, moderate or severe according to the number of symptoms present.[6]

**TABLE 26.1** Symptoms contributing to a diagnosis of depressive disorder

| Symptoms comparable to those in adults | Symptoms more likely to occur in adolescents or children |
|---|---|
| Low mood for most of the time | Bouts of low mood |
| Tearfulness | Irritability (easily annoyed or provoked) |
| Loss of confidence or self-esteem | Overall anxiety |
| A reduced ability to enjoy anything | Separation anxiety (which may present as school refusal) |
| A reduced ability to think or concentrate | |
| Spending less time with friends | Decline in school work |
| Guilt or self-reproach (out of proportion) | Complaints of boredom |
| A variety of physical symptoms | Specific physical symptoms (pains in bones, joints or head) |
| Reduced quality of sleep | |
| Waking up tired | Sleeping more (instead of less) |
| Change in appetite with corresponding weight change | Middle insomnia |
| | Antisocial behaviour – especially in boys |
| Becoming agitated or sluggish | Substance misuse |
| Recurrent thoughts of death or suicide | Running away from home |
| Self-harm | |

Depression may be accompanied by *psychotic symptoms*, such as auditory or visual hallucinations or delusions, often with a persecutory flavour (*see* Chapter 41 on Imaginary Friends, Voices and Psychosis). Sometimes, the young person talks about feeling that people are looking at him or talking about him, even though he knows they are not (*ideas of reference* rather than delusions). Ideas of reference are common in substance misuse, particularly with cannabis. The presence of psychotic symptoms usually requires further assessment in specialist CAMHS or an early intervention in psychosis service, depending on how local referral pathways are constructed. In addition to depressive disorder and substance misuse, other possibilities include schizophrenia or bipolar disorder, which may be difficult to distinguish in the early stages.

### Bipolar disorder

Manic depression (bipolar disorder) in young people is hard to assess.[7,8] To simplify somewhat, standard definitions require a distinct episode of elevated mood with three concurrent features from a list that includes various features of mania, especially euphoria or grandiosity (others are listed later in this paragraph). Some young people however have episodes that do not last the requisite four days (some may have 'rapid cycling' – frequent up-and-down changes of mood); while others have a baseline presence of 'manic-like symptoms', dominated by irritability rather than euphoria, without clear episodes. Young people in the second group often have a diagnosis of ADHD (*see* Chapter 31) or oppositional defiant disorder (*see* Chapter 30) – with symptoms in addition to irritability such as: social disinhibition, recklessness, intrusiveness, insensitivity, distractibility, restlessness, agitation, a decreased need for sleep, talkativeness, or racing thoughts. Some at least of the first group (those with episodes lasting less than four days) seem to develop strict bipolar disorder if followed for long enough. Most of the second group (those with baseline levels of manic-like or ADHD symptoms) probably do not, although, just to add to the confusion, they may be more at risk of developing depressive disorder, particular if they tend to be intermittently sad or angry. Transatlantic differences are particularly marked in relation to the frequency of diagnosis of bipolar disorder: a European perspective is that over-diagnosis of a bipolar tendency may inappropriately encourage the use in children of the sort of medications used to treat adult bipolar disorder.[9] From a clinical point of view, it is probably best not to make a firm diagnosis (or accept someone else's diagnosis) of bipolar disorder without definite out-of-character episodes of elevated mood (or irritability) combined with other manic features.[10] This in any case is a task for specialist CAMHS.

## ASSESSMENT
### Possible questions

To work out if a young person is depressed, the ideal is to **see her on her own** as well as seeing her carers – either together with her or separately or both. The parents may be largely unaware of how their teenager is feeling. As in more general interviews, ask open questions first, followed by questions that are more specific. Table 26.2 shows a list of possible questions to ask, but of course the exact questions depend on the individual, the context and the answers given to previous questions.

The **time pattern** of adolescent depression is different from adults. Mood is characteristically very variable – less pervasive than in adults. A depressed adolescent may be in the depths of despair one moment, and enjoying a social outing with friends an hour later. The fact that she can still enjoy certain aspects of her life does not exclude a depressive disorder. In adults, diagnostic criteria demand a duration of symptoms of at least two weeks. In adolescents, it is probably wiser to wait until mood and other changes have persisted for four weeks before making a diagnosis.

Do not be frightened to ask about **suicidal ideas** or intent (*see* sixth column of Table 26.2): there is no evidence that this affects the risk of suicidal actions. On the contrary, the young person may be relieved at sharing such ideas and feelings. A general question about feeling like dying can be followed by more specific questions about concrete plans.

Many of these questions may be met with **a shrug of the shoulders**, a 'Don't know …' or no answer at all. This seems to be more common in boys, who are often less adept at putting feelings into words. Boys are probably less likely to get to see a professional anyway, and depression in boys tends to be under-diagnosed. Faced with this, you may arrange either to see the young person again, or make a referral to a primary mental health worker or specialist CAMHS. However, such recalcitrance suggests the young person may not accept or comply with an onward referral. Another way of dealing with the repeated shoulder-shrug is to make guesses about the young person's feelings, and ask her to nod or shake her head so you can

**TABLE 26.2** Some questions that could be asked in the assessment of depression

| Exploratory | About specific features of depression | | | | About suicidal intent | If you seem to be getting nowhere |
|---|---|---|---|---|---|---|
| | Emotional | Cognitive | Behavioural | Biological | | |
| How have you been feeling recently? | Have you been feeling as happy as usual/ sadder than usual/ down-in the dumps recently? | How do you feel about yourself at the moment? | Are you currently more active or less active than usual? | What time do you go to bed? | Having you been feeling so low that you have thought about dying? | It seems like you feel pretty fed-up with this whole situation, including having to see me? |
| What sort of things do you enjoy doing at the moment? | What are you feeling like inside? | What sort of things are you interested in at present? | Are you seeing as much as you would like of your friends? | What time do you get off to sleep? | Have you thought you might be better off dead? | Maybe you are fed-up with life in general? |
| How have you been getting on with your friends recently? | Do you think you've been getting cross more than usual recently? | How are you managing to concentrate at school? | Have you done anything to harm yourself? | What happens in between? | Have you ever thought about killing yourself? | Maybe it feels like no-one could possibly understand how you feel, so there's not much point in trying to explain it? |
| How have you been getting on at school/college recently? | Are you crying a lot – or finding it difficult to cry? | What do you feel about the future? | If so, how does this make you feel? | Do you wake up after you have gone to sleep? How many times? How long does it take you to get back to sleep? | What have you thought of doing to yourself? | |

How have you
been getting on
with your family
recently?

Is there anything
you feel guilty
about?

Have you run
away from home?

What do you feel
like when you
wake up at the
start of your day?
Refreshed or
exhausted?

Have you been
eating more or
less than usual
recently?

Do you ever
binge eat?

Do you know
anyone (relative/
friend/public
figure) who has
killed herself?

tell whether your wild speculations are right or wrong. You can ask questions such as those in the last column of Table 26.2.

A simple way of trying to gauge the severity of the problem is *scaling*: ask the young person to rate the severity of her depression on a scale of zero to 10, where 10 is as happy as possible and zero is the unhappiest she could be. This can be repeated at intervals to assess progress (or lack of it). Rating scales that have been developed for research can also be used clinically to assess the level of depression and response to treatment: two such scales that are available on the Internet without significant copyright restrictions are the Mood and Feelings Questionnaire,[11] developed specifically for young people, and the Beck Depression Inventory[12] – which, although designed for adults, may be suitable for those aged 15 years and over. These may sometimes help stimulate discussion in those who are initially reluctant to talk about themselves.

Try to come to a decision about whether the constellation of depressive symptoms is present and is affecting the young person's functioning. Alternative explanations may include sadness appropriate to circumstances, anxiety, or substance misuse – but any of these may co-exist with a depressive disorder – and often do.

### Contributory factors

As with young people who harm themselves, there may be concealed precipitating factors, such as sexual abuse or rape, family relationship difficulties or bullying at school. It is particularly important to enquire about losses, some of which may not be obvious. For instance, the death of a pet may be a major life event for a young person, as may moving house and school, the loss of close friends or relatives through house moves, or the death of a grandparent – however expected this might be. A family history of depressive disorder, bipolar disorder or alcoholism predisposes to adolescent depression. Recreational drugs or alcohol may be taken to improve mood, but will generally have the opposite effect. The case example in Box 26.2 is expanded in Table 26.3 to include contributory factors that emerge in the 14-year-old girl's second assessment (after her overdose).

### MANAGEMENT

Treatment should be tailored to the individual child, young person or family, and may include social, psychological and pharmacological components. It is likely to involve not only the young person but also her family and potentially other professionals who already have contact with her, such as those at her school.

### Psychoeducation

A useful starting point is to obtain the young person's consent to explain to her parents, preferably in her presence, how she is feeling. This can lead on to a discussion of the nature of depression, perhaps backed up by some of the resources below. Consider a book prescription if you have a scheme operating in your area. Depending on the level of curiosity within the family, it may be worth trying to define

**TABLE 26.3** Four-P grid applied to Case Example in Box 26.2

|  | Biological | Psychological | Social |
| --- | --- | --- | --- |
| **Predisposing** (Vulnerability factors) | Paternal grandfather (who never left India) had what sounds as if it might have been bipolar disorder | High achiever: disappointed if she doesn't achieve the high standards she sets herself | High family expectations |
| **Precipitating** (Trigger factors) |  | Mother lost her job two months ago Pet rabbit died four months ago | Conflict with friends (possibly a result rather than a cause – could be both) |
| **Perpetuating** (Maintaining factors) |  | Too easily able to pretend she is 'fine' when actually she is not Elder and younger brothers tease her without realising it actually hurts her | Wants to protect others around her, so gets everyone else to confide in her, but herself confides in no one |
| **Protective** (Resilience) | Appears to have high intelligence and be above average academically | Capable of reflection and insight | Supportive, caring parents |

depression, discussing its causes; discussing what may happen if nothing is done; and looking at the relative merits of employing or not employing different components of treatment.

## Social interventions

It may or may not be relatively straightforward to address any sources of distress, such as bullying, and remove opportunities for self-harm, such as paracetamol lying around the house. Practical help with exam stress or social activities should be relatively easy to organise.

Conflicts arising within the family may require some form of *family work* to resolve; sometimes a single family discussion may be enough. Guidelines for brief family work include: managing high expectations, taking a problem-solving approach (*see* below), planning positive interactions between family members, and encouraging parents to provide plentiful positive reinforcement for any small steps forward. Providing support for parents is important, as is identifying depression in either parent and making every effort to get it adequately treated.[13] Once recovery has begun, it is worth involving the family in planning what to do if there is a relapse.

## Psychological interventions

*Talking about feelings and sources of worry* can be helpful, whomever it is with. Many young people prefer to talk to friends rather than to a professional, and some may be able to confide in their parents. Alternatives include sympathetic staff at school, youth workers, other trusted adults – from within or outside the family – a practice counsellor, primary mental health worker or team member in specialist CAMHS. The research seems to suggest that a complete package of support is as important as the training of the professional or the treatment model she uses. For instance, cognitive behavioural therapy, which aims to make emotions more positive by encouraging positive thoughts[14] may be no more effective than standard treatment,[15] and is probably more effective if combined with medication;[16,17] and interpersonal therapy, which focuses on relationships, role conflicts and grief.[18] This implies that the lack of widespread availability of specialised treatments such as cognitive-behavioural therapy and interpersonal therapy may not matter, since talking through the issues that the young person chooses to discuss, using an empathic reflective approach, may be just as effective.[19] This should ideally be combined with practical interventions and continuing professional support.

## Medication

Clinical practice suggests that antidepressants make depressive disorder better. This may be partly due to a placebo effect, but research suggests that they are almost twice as effective as placebo.[20] Clinical guidelines recommend starting a selective serotonin reuptake inhibitor such as fluoxetine as part of the initial treatment for severe depression (preferably in conjunction with some talking treatment) and after a period of psychological treatment in moderate depression.[21] There has been much debate about an increase in suicidal thoughts and self-harm in the few weeks after starting medication, an effect that seems to be more likely in adolescents than adults.[22] It seems however that the risk of completed suicide is greater if the depression is *not* treated with everything available, including medication: the benefits of antidepressants appear to be much greater than the risks from suicidal ideas or attempts.[23]

Alternatives to fluoxetine include sertraline, citalopram or mirtazapine. Parents may sometimes ask for St John's Wort, thinking it must be safe because it is herbal. In fact, the active ingredient may be very similar to selective serotonin reuptake inhibitors, the dose is not standardised between different preparations, and it can interact with other medicines, importantly reducing the efficacy of the oral contraceptive pill – so it is not recommended for adolescents.[24]

## Other elements of a successful treatment package

It is important to adopt a ***collaborative approach*** between professional and young person. Any help provided is likely to be more effective if the young person feels she has helped to decide what she will do to get better and has some ownership of the management plan.

Look for any ***protective factors*** in the young person's temperament or situation, and build upon these. Help parents also to identify the young person's strengths and positive attributes.

*Activity scheduling* involves planning a timetable of positive activities that can distract the young person from depressive ruminations and help her begin to establish a routine of physical and mental exercise and social contact. Find out what she enjoys and use this as a basis for a jointly constructed plan, setting small incremental goals. This may involve reinstating previously enjoyed activities as well as thinking up new ones. Be aware that the inertia and avoidance characteristic of a depressive disorder will make this difficult, and ensure that self-reward, parental praise and professional encouragement is available for every small step forward.

**BOX 26.4** Case Example

Cynthia, aged 15 years, is working on her depression with her school counsellor. They have involved her teachers in reducing the number of GCSEs she will take and renegotiating coursework deadlines. Now they agree to work on activity scheduling. They both know that Cynthia's GCSE work is a priority, but the counsellor emphasizes that Cynthia must build pleasurable activities into her daily routine, to help improve her mood and concentration.

They discuss what Cynthia found enjoyable before she was depressed. The list includes swimming, hanging out with friends and horse-riding: Cynthia has gradually stopped doing all these things. She agrees to restart swimming once a week after school, and is able to arrange for a friend to join her with this. The counsellor is not sure that unstructured 'hanging out' is going to be very helpful, but suggests that Cynthia should ask her parents to reward her with a weekend horse-riding lesson every week that she meets a (revised) coursework deadline; again, Cynthia is able to enrol one of her long-standing friends in this.

This proves to be a good beginning to re-establishing a weekly routine of activities and social contact, which contributes to an improvement in Cynthia's concentration and mood.

*Sleep hygiene* may be helpful: see the adolescent section of Chapter 17 on Sleep Problems.

*Self-care* may be impaired in depression. As well as the progressive abandonment of sleep routines, washing and eating routines may also deteriorate. Reinstating these will add to the benefits of activity scheduling in providing a structure to each day. Regular *exercise* may be important: a suggested target is 45 minutes to one hour three times per week.[25] Similarly, establishing a regular *diet* may contribute to recovery: there is emerging evidence of the impact of dietary inadequacy on mood[26] (*See also* Chapter 44 on Diet and Exercise).

*Problem-solving* may be an important component of successful psychological therapy for adolescents.[27] It can be taught relatively easily, by working on particular issues of concern to the young person. This is described in Chapter 13 on Behaviour Management; it can be summarised by the following five components.

➤ Define the problem. How would I know if things were better? What goals would it be realistic to aim for?

➤ Brainstorm solutions. What are some plans that we could try?

➤ Evaluate consequences. What is the best plan? What is the best compromise between an ideal outcome and an achievable outcome?

➤ Implementation. Am I using my plan?

➤ Evaluating the outcome and revising the plan. How did I do?

**BOX 26.5** Case Example

Fergus is 16 years old when he splits up with Lucy, his girlfriend of two years, and becomes depressed. Every time he sees Lucy he feels despondent and discarded. He is desperate to see her, but realizes that seeing her makes him feel worse. If he tries to be 'just friends' with her, he finds that Lucy soon says something that makes him very angry, so that he shouts at her, and she rejects him all over again.

The professional who is helping Fergus recover from his depression discusses this with him as a problem to be solved.

*First,* they define the problem: he can't be with Lucy or without her. She matters so much to him that even thinking about her evokes powerful emotions, and she is so under his skin that he cannot be anywhere near her without revealing these emotions. Fergus sets as his initial goal being more able to tolerate managing without Lucy.

*Second,* they brainstorm solutions. These include:

1 not seeing or talking to Lucy at all
2 writing her a letter every night but not sending it
3 emigrating to Australia
4 joining the army
5 going to a local sixth-form college so that he doesn't have to be at the same school as Lucy
6 writing a private dairy of how he feels
7 writing a blog on Facebook of how he feels
8 going somewhere far away from anyone once a week and shouting and screaming as loudly as he can
9 talking to a male friend about how impossible girls are to deal with.

*Third,* they discuss each of these possibilities, and Fergus decides to try numbers one, two, eight and nine.

*Fourth,* Fergus puts these suggestions into action.

*Fifth,* when he reviews these after four weeks, he reports as follows. The shouting and screaming made him feel better the first time, but from the third time onwards it seemed to make him feel more churned up inside, so he has stopped this. Talking to a male friend also helped the first couple of times, but then seemed to make him ruminate painfully on Lucy – so he has stopped this too. Writing letters to Lucy has definitely helped, he thinks probably more than a diary or blog would have, and it was a wise decision not to send them (they will remain private). Fergus no longer needs to do this every night, but will continue as often as he feels the need. Not seeing or talking to Lucy has been exceedingly difficult, and he has seen her several times at school, but walked in the opposite direction. He has made enquiries about changing to the sixth-form college (solution five), and has discovered that this will be relatively easy after his GCSEs, providing he gets good enough grades, so he is going to work towards this, despite the decline in academic performance he has noticed recently. He no longer feels like emigrating to Australia, or joining the army 'in order to get blown up by a roadside bomb in Afghanistan': in fact, his depression is beginning to get better.

As can be seen from this case example, young people can learn as much from solutions that do not work as ones that do.

It is often a central task for the professional to help the young person put feelings into words. This may mean developing together a vocabulary for describing feelings. It can be called *affective education*. Feelings can then be linked to activities or relationships or losses or memories or habits of thinking.

*Mood monitoring* using the 1–10 scale mentioned earlier can be very useful as a marker of progress and a stimulus to self-reflection. Alternatively, you can use a depression rating scale suitable for young people, such as the two mentioned above.

Training in *social skills* may be important. Components of this can include the following.[28]

➤ How to be assertive rather than aggressive – proactive rather than passive.
➤ How to use 'I' statements to express feelings rather than sounding critical of others. This builds on the affective education described above, developing it into an interpersonal skill.
➤ Active listening and reflecting.
➤ How to start a conversation and continue it. How to join groups when you don't feel a part of them.
➤ Accurate communication with others, rather than for instance keeping everything to yourself, or expecting others to understand your point of view without explaining it to them.
➤ Compromise: how to negotiate a solution that meets others halfway and resolve conflicts once they develop.
➤ Family communication: reducing blame and name-calling, clearly identifying things that you want or problems that you experience, increasing trust and using the above listening and communication skills within the family.

*Involving the school* may be necessary to ensure continued attendance or gradually reinstate this if lapsed, deal with any peer conflicts, make allowances for impaired concentration, address missed deadlines for coursework, reduce the number of exams taken if appropriate, and provide extra help if required, for instance with study skills or specific learning difficulties (*see* Case Example in Box 26.4). An adolescent may initially be reluctant to allow staff at school to know how she is feeling, and this must be respected, but it is worth persevering until she can see that there are ways of improving things at school – but only if her teachers understand what she is going through.

Attention to any **comorbid problems** may be very important, such as anxiety or ADHD.

**BOX 26.6** Case Example

In the last two years, Mia, aged 15 years, has been diagnosed with Crohn's disease and diabetes. She has had repeated hospital admissions, mainly for exacerbations of her Crohn's disease, and much time off school. She has also had to give up her dance and performing arts activities, as she cannot attend regularly. Her consultant paediatrician arranges for Mia to see the paediatric psychologist, as he is concerned about her low mood and poor sleep. During Mia's last two admissions for Crohn's disease flare-ups, the ward staff have observed significant tension and repeated arguments between Mia and her mother, often about her diet.

The psychologist and Mia meet a number of times; they explore Mia's fluctuating mood and the factors that improve or worsen it. From this it becomes clear that Mia feels more and more peripheral amongst those who used to be her friends because of her increasing withdrawal from school and the activities she used to enjoy. This has led her to rely more and more on her mother, which at times Mia greatly resents. Mia explains that when she is unwell she is grateful for her mother's help and practical support, but at other times she wants to be as independent as possible. Mia experiences her mother treating her like a much younger child and sees this as a basis for many of their arguments.

The goals Mia agrees to work on are:

- to be able to manage her diet by herself
- to be able to make decisions regarding her education and what subjects she will study
- to persuade her mother to respect her need for age-appropriate social contact – in Mia's words: 'to be able to stay out as late as my friends'.

The psychologist helps Mia and her mother learn how to discuss difficult issues together, such as giving Mia more independence and autonomy. This involves teaching Mia how to express her feelings in a non-blaming way using 'I' statements and also the skills of problem-solving and compromise. Mia and the psychologist spend time discussing how to make interactions with her mother a 'win-win' situation rather than 'win-lose' or 'lose-lose'.

Together they discuss activity scheduling and look at planning which activities Mia can do when she is well and which when she is unwell, focusing particularly on those that give her opportunities for social contact. Interestingly, Mia chooses some activities that she used to do with her mother that have lapsed due to the recent conflict, such as trips to the family allotment, crochet and needlework. The psychologist supports Mia and her mother in talking to her Head of Year at school.

Over the next few months, Mia's mood gradually stabilises without the need for antidepressant medication. Her social contact with peers and her relationship with her mother both improve gradually. Mia is also able to organise a reduced timetable at school, enabling her to focus on five achievable GCSEs – which is enough for the art and design course she hopes to get into at sixth-form college.

## REFERRAL

Should *all* depressed adolescents be referred to a specialist service? Referral to specialist CAMHS is clearly indicated if there is evidence of suicidal intent, psychotic experiences or a pattern of up-and-down mood. A close family history of depression, alcoholism, bipolar disorder or schizophrenia should also prompt referral. If a young person or her parents wants a trial of antidepressants, she will usually need to see a child and adolescent psychiatrist, as most general practitioners have become understandably reluctant to prescribe for under-18s because of the concern about increasing suicidal ideas and the 2005 NICE guidelines: some may nevertheless be prepared to prescribe with telephone support from a specialist.[29]

**BOX 26.7** Alarm Bells in the assessment of adolescent depression: indications for referral

Suicidal ideas accompanied by clearly thought-out plans
Psychotic experiences including hallucinations, delusions or ideas of reference, even if drug use seems a likely explanation
A clearly repeated pattern of up-and-down mood, however short or long the ups or downs or gaps
A close family history of depression, alcoholism, bipolar disorder or schizophrenia

Many other cases may be manageable by a variety of professionals in the community without specialist referral, but some will need onward referral if concerns emerge or if clear progress is not made.

**BOX 26.8** Practice Points for the management of depressive disorder

Children and adolescents can develop a syndrome of depression that shares many similarities with the adult equivalent.
    Assessment should include an exploration of contributing factors.
    Ask specifically about suicidal intent and plans.
    Management may involve:
- talking interventions
- family interventions
- school interventions
- medication.

## RESOURCES
### Websites for young people or their parents
- Royal College of Psychiatrists leaflets. London: Royal College of Psychiatrists; 2009.
- www.rcpsych.ac.uk/mentalhealthinfoforall/youngpeople.aspx
- **Youth in Mind**: This website provides help for stressed children and teenagers and those who care for them. www.youthinmind.com
- **Depression in Teenagers**: This website is aimed at teenagers and gives useful advice about depression and its treatment. www.depressioninteenagers.co.uk
- **Black Dog Institute:** This website gives useful information on depression for parents and young people. www.blackdoginstitute.org.au/public/depression/inteenagersyoungadults.cfm

### Books for young people or their parents
- Fitzpatrick C, Sharry J. *Coping with Depression: a guide for parents*. Chichester and Oxford: Wiley-Blackwell; 2004.
- Chilman-Blair K, Deloache S. What's Up with James? Medikidz explain depression. London: Medikidz Publishing; 2010.
- Garland J. *Depression Is the Pits, But I'm Getting Better: a guide for adolescents*. Washington DC: Magination Press (American Psychological Association); 1997.
  A clear and user-friendly guide that will be helpful to anyone suffering from depression.
- Graham PJ, Hughes C. *So Young, So Sad, So Listen*. 2nd ed. Gaskell; London: 2005.
  This book is very easy to read and packed with useful information.
- Stilwell V, Roche C. *Living with a Stranger*. London: Gaskell (Royal College of Psychiatrists); 1997.
  This book is intended for carers of all ages who live with someone suffering from depression.

### Resources for healthcare professionals
- The Royal College of General Practitioners has guidance on the management of adolescent depression in primary care: www.rcgp.org.uk/default.aspx?page=6954

## REFERENCES
1 Thapar A, Collishaw S, Potter R, *et al*. Managing and preventing depression in adolescents. *BMJ*. 2010 Jan 22; **340**: 254–8.
2 Ibid.
3 Ibid.
4 Egger HL, Costello EJ, Erkanli A, *et al*. Somatic complaints and psychopathology in children and adolescents: stomach aches, musculoskeletal pains, and headaches. *J Am Acad Child Adolesc Psychiatry*. 1999; **38**(7): 852–60.
5 Egger HL, Angold A, Costello EJ. Headaches and psychopathology in children and adolescents. *J Am Acad Child Adolesc Psychiatry*. 1998; **37**(9): 951–8.
6 National Institute for Health and Clinical Excellence. *Depression in children and young people: identification and management in primary, community and secondary care*. NICE Clinical Guideline number 28. London: NICE; 2005. Available at: http://guidance.nice.org.uk/CG28/niceguidance/pdf/English (accessed 29 March 2011).
7 Baroni A, Lunsford JR, Luckenbaugh DA, *et al*. Practitioner Review: The assessment of bipolar disorder in children and adolescents. *Journal of Child Psychology and Psychiatry*. 2009; **50**(3): 203–15.

8 Leibenluft E, Rich BA. Pediatric Bipolar Disorder. *Annual Review of Clinical Psychology.* 2008; **4**: 163–87. Available at: http://focus.psychiatryonline.org/cgi/reprint/6/3/331 (accessed 29 March 2011).

9 National Institute for Health and Clinical Excellence. *Bipolar disorder: the management of bipolar disorder in adults, children and adolescents in primary and secondary care.* NICE Clinical Guideline number 38. London: NICE; 2006. Full guideline: appendix 19; p. 526). Available at: http://guidance.nice.org.uk/CG38 (accessed 29 March 2011).

10 Baroni, op. cit.

11 http://devepi.duhs.duke.edu/mfq.html gives information about the Mood and Feelings Questionnaire, which can be downloaded free from this site.

12 www.ibogaine.desk.nl/graphics/3639b1c_23.pdf

13 Garber J, Clarke GN, Weersing V, *et al.* Prevention of depression in at-risk adolescents: a randomized controlled trial. *JAMA.* 2009; **301**(21): 2215–24.

14 Stallard P. *Think Good – Feel Good: a cognitive behaviour therapy workbook for children and young people.* Oxford: Wiley-Blackwell; 2002.

15 Goodyer I, Dubicka B, Wilkinson P, *et al.* Selective serotonin reuptake inhibitors (SSRIs) and routine specialist care with and without cognitive behaviour therapy in adolescents with major depression: randomised controlled trial. *BMJ.* 2007; **335**: 142.

16 Treatment for Adolescents with Depression Study (TADS) Team. The treatment for adolescents with depression study (TADS): outcomes over 1 year of naturalistic follow-up. *Am J Psychiatry.* 2009; **166**: 1141–9.

17 Brent D, Emslie G, Clarke G, *et al.* Switching to another SSRI or to venlafaxine with or without cognitive behavioral therapy for adolescents with SSRI-resistant depression: the TORDIA randomized controlled trial. *JAMA.* 2008; **299**(8): 901–13.

18 Mufson L, Weissman MM, Moreau D, *et al.* Efficacy of interpersonal psychotherapy for depressed adolescents. *Archives of General Psychiatry.* 1999; **56**(6): 573–9.

19 Goodyer, op. cit.

20 Thapar, op. cit. p. 255.

21 National Institute for Health and Clinical Excellence, op. cit.

22 Barbui C, Esposito E, Cipriani A. Selective serotonin reuptake inhibitors and risk of suicide: a systematic review of observational studies. *Canadian Medical Association Journal.* 2009; **180**(3): 291–7.

23 Bridge JA, Iyengar S, Salary CB, *et al.* Clinical response and risk for reported suicidal ideation and suicide attempts in pediatric antidepressant treatment: a meta-analysis of randomized controlled trials. *JAMA.* 2007; **297**(15): 1683–96.

24 National Institute for Health and Clinical Excellence, op. cit.

25 Ibid.

26 Fulkerson JA, Sherwood NE, Perry CL, *et al.* Depressive symptoms and adolescent eating and health behaviors: a multifaceted view in a population-based sample. *Prev Med.* 2004; **38**(6): 865–75.

27 Kennard BD, Clarke GN, Weersing VR, *et al.* Effective components of TORDIA cognitive-behavioral therapy for adolescent depression: preliminary findings. *J Consult Clin Psychol.* 2009; **77**(6): 1033–41.

28 Kennard, op. cit.

29 National Institute for Health and Clinical Excellence, op. cit.

# CHAPTER 27

# Self-harm

## INTRODUCTION

### Definition and prevalence

Self-harm can be defined as 'self-poisoning or injury, irrespective of the purpose of the act'.[1] There has been a trend in the UK recently to drop the word 'deliberate' in front of self-harm, and to abandon the term 'attempted suicide', on the grounds that the person's intention is not always clear. How, for instance, do we understand a young person who is 'playing around' with some form of self-harm, and appears to inadvertently end his own life? The Case Example in Box 27.1 is a very tragic example of this (except that it could be argued that it is not even an instance of self-harm). The trend on the opposite side of the Atlantic is different, in that self-harm is split into two groups: 'non-suicidal self-injury' and 'suicidal self-injury'.

**BOX 27.1** Case Example

> Leticia, aged 10 years, is alone in her shared bedroom, while her parents and seven-year-old brother, Jeff, are downstairs. Their parents ask Jeff what Leticia was doing when he left her to come downstairs. He says that she found a piece of rope on her way back from school and was playing with it in their bedroom. Their father goes up to investigate, and finds Leticia hanging from the top rung of the bunk bed, dead.
>
> No one in Leticia's family knows of any reason why she might want to kill herself. As far as everyone is aware, Leticia is perfectly happy and enjoying school. Her parents are offered an appointment with a family therapist to discuss how they might cope with their grief, but decline it. The coroner records a verdict of accidental death.

In an international study of the prevalence of self-harm, young people aged 14–17 years were asked the question: 'Have you ever deliberately taken an overdose, e.g. of pills or other medication, or tried to harm yourself in some other way (such as cut yourself)?'[2] The results showed a prevalence of self-harm in the preceding year of about 9% in girls and 3% in boys. Only 12% of these presented to hospital

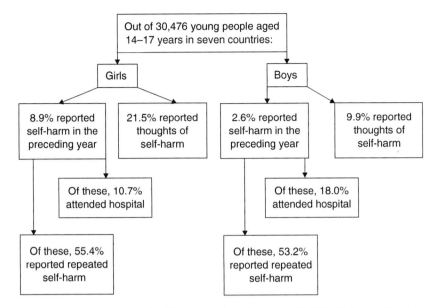

**FIGURE 27.1** Epidemiology of self-harm, taken from the CASE (Child and Adolescent Self-harm in Europe) Study

(7% of cutters and 18% of those who overdosed), although 75% told someone else. Approximately half reported repeated self-harm. *Thoughts of self-harm* occurred in an additional 22% of girls and 10% of boys. (*See* Figure 27.1 for more exact figures.) *Methods* described by the young people surveyed who had done something to themselves included:

➤ self-cutting
➤ hanging or strangulation
➤ suffocation
➤ jumping or throwing self
➤ electrocution
➤ self-battery
➤ alcohol
➤ burning
➤ inhalation/sniffing
➤ starvation
➤ stopping of medication
➤ shooting
➤ drowning
➤ freezing
➤ overdose
➤ consuming a recreational drug when regarded as self-harm by the young person himself
➤ swallowing a non-ingestible substance or object.

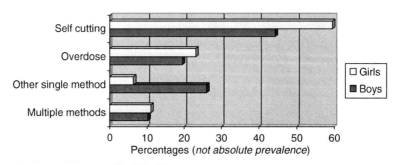

**FIGURE 27.2** Self-harm categories from the CASE (Child and Adolescent Self-harm in Europe) Study

These methods were grouped into four categories: cutting, overdosing, other single methods and multiple methods. The relative frequencies of these for boys and girls are shown in Figure 27.2 (as percentages, not absolute prevalence).

In school-age adolescents, **self-cutting** tends to be superficial and of mainly cosmetic importance – in contrast to adults, who may cut deeply and damage tendons or nerves. The left forearm is a common site, but any accessible part of the body can be incised, with a variety of sharp objects. Cutting is more likely to be impulsive than overdosing, and less likely to be directed towards dying.[3]

The significance of the type of self-harm also varies in terms of how likely an attempt is to be followed by successful suicide. Extrapolating from an adult population study in Sweden,[4] the most worrying attempts are hanging, drowning, jumping and firearm use, in that order.

### Risk factors

In any one case, it is likely there will be several risk factors combined. Risk factors could be divided into groups in several ways, for instance using the four-P grid (*see* Chapter 6 on Resilience and Risk), or looking at the impact of culture, parents and friends on what leads to self-harm, the function it serves and the aftermath. Factors making self-harm more or less likely, and which are therefore worth looking out for in any assessment, include the following.[5,6]

➤ **Gender** – Girls are more likely to self-harm or have thoughts of self-harm than boys (*see* Figure 27.1 for comparative prevalence rates); but boys are more likely to complete suicide.

➤ **Age** – The main age for self-harm in both boys and girls seems to be from 14–18 years. It occurs less commonly in 12–14 year olds, and even less often below 12 years.[7] The reason for the dramatic increase at 14 years may be partly due to the increased pressures of schoolwork at this age, as discussed below, but is likely to be due also to other factors, such as increasing concern about identity, social and sexual pressures and experimentation with risk-taking behaviours (*see* Chapter 4 on Adolescence).

➤ *Ethnicity* – Clear, consistent patterns are difficult to find.[8] Self-harm may be less common in cohesive and sizable communities, but more common in ethnic minorities who form a small proportion of the local population. Conflict between the culture of origin and the adopted culture may increase the risk of self-harm, particularly if it results in family tensions.

➤ *Socioeconomic deprivation* seems not to increase the risk of self-harm for under-18s, in contrast to over-18s, for whom self-harm is commoner in lower socioeconomic groups.

➤ *Family factors* – Poor communication within the family may make it more difficult for the young person to communicate her distress verbally than by her actions. Family harmony and cohesion reduce the risk of self-harm. Lack of parental support, criticism from parents, conflict between the young person and her parents, and conflict between parents all seem to increase the risk of self-harm. Separation and divorce also seem to be associated with self-harm, perhaps mainly because of the conflict involved. The self-harm risk seems to be more increased in boys than in girls when not having their biological father living in the home.[9] Exposure to nonfatal suicidal behaviours in family members makes deliberate self-harm more likely.[10]

➤ *Poor problem-solving abilities* – If the most effective coping strategy for a young person is to self-harm, then something is likely to be wrong either with the alternatives open to her or with her ability to generate alternative solutions.[11,12] Problem-solving is a skill that has to be learnt, can readily be taught, but is deficient in a number of mental health presentations (including not only self-harm but also conduct disorder and depression).

➤ *Impulsivity* – Particularly in girls; this may be a personality trait, a reflection of feelings such as hopelessness, or part of a deficiency in problem-solving skills. The more the impulsivity, the less the seriousness of the suicidal intent.

**BOX 27.2** Case Example

From the age of 15–16 years, Olivia presents to hospital with recurrent, impulsive small overdoses of whatever tablets she can find. These often include paracetomol. After her ninth overdose, she develops nausea and jaundice, and is found to have paracetomol-induced liver damage. Fortunately, she recovers completely with supportive medical management. She does not take any further overdoses.

➤ *Hopelessness* – This can occur independently from depression, or as part of a constellation of depressive symptoms. The more the hopelessness, the more serious the suicidal intent.

➤ *Low self-esteem* – This also can occur independently from depression, or as part of a constellation of depressive symptoms.

➤ Other symptoms of *depression* may apply (*see* Chapter 26 on Depression for more details).

**BOX 27.3** Case Example

A health visitor carries out a routine home visit to see Gurpreet, a six-month-old baby. She is alarmed when the baby's mother tells her that Gurpreet's 14-year-old half-brother Steven has just admitted to taking a whole packet of 16 paracetomol the previous week. This seems to have followed an argument between Steven and his father.

The health visitor telephones the primary mental health worker for advice – which is that Steven's general practitioner should be asked to see him as soon as possible, to assess what else is going on and whether there is any ongoing risk. Steven is seen at the end of evening surgery the same day.

Steven admits to his general practitioner that he is disappointed the overdose did not achieve more: initially he felt better, but now he feels just as bad. He has been feeling low in mood for two to three months. He acknowledges being angry with his father for letting him down about promised contact and presents, neither of which materialise. He is struggling with his Year 10 schoolwork and having difficulty maintaining his concentration and motivation. He has stopped going to his weekend football practice and league games. He finds most of his social life much more difficult to enjoy than it used to be. He has been taking two to three hours to get to sleep, and wakes two or three times each night, taking at least half an hour to get back to sleep.

In view of the multiple features of depression and the risk of further overdose, the general practitioner makes an urgent referral to specialist CAMHS. Steven is assessed the following week and offered regular appointments for talking treatment. He finds he gets on better with this than he expected. After six weeks, there is slight improvement; he and his mother are asked if they want an appointment with a psychiatrist to discuss possible medication. Steven is not sure, but his mother is very much against medication, so he agrees to persevere with the talking treatment. Both parents are offered an appointment to discuss the possibility of family work, but Steven's father opts out of this.

After allowing discussion between his therapist and his school Head of Year, Steven is helped to rationalise his workload and is allowed to drop some of his planned GCSE subjects, on condition that he uses the free periods in school to catch up on his coursework. After six months of weekly individual sessions, Steven feels more able to enjoy the company of his friends. He has been able to explore with his therapist (amongst other themes) how he feels unloved and undervalued by his father. He continues to improve with fortnightly sessions for the next three months, and remains much better at one final session a year after his overdose.

➤ *Anxiety*, including social anxiety, may be a factor (but many features of anxiety may overlap with the features of depression in adolescence).
➤ *Eating disorders* – Bulimia especially is associated with self-harm (*see* Chapter 28 on Eating Disorders).
➤ *Substance misuse*
  — There seems to be a strong link between use of non-prescribed illicit substances and self-harm.

— There is a similarly strong association between amount of *alcohol* use and self-harm.

— There is also a relationship between smoking *cigarettes* and self-harm. This may be a reflection of some common factors leading to both.

➤ *Schoolwork-related stresses* can often be important. Common factors such as low self-esteem, lack of encouragement at home or depressive symptoms may contribute to both difficulties keeping up with schoolwork and self-harm. The authors' experience is that self-harm becomes much commoner from the beginning of Year 10 at school, which is the start of the build-up to GCSEs and the pressure associated with this.

**BOX 27.4** Case Example

Gloria takes her first overdose on the way to school at age 14. Later in the day she begins to experience abdominal cramps, and tells her best friend, who tells their Head of Year, who calls an ambulance.

It emerges that Gloria is behind with her GCSE coursework and is struggling to cope. She has felt unable to tell anyone in her family or the teachers at school, whom she experiences as putting a lot of pressure on her to achieve good results in coursework. Although her friends also feel under pressure, she thinks she is the only one who is finding it all so difficult.

➤ *Peer relationships* – Having friends to confide in may offer a channel for communication that serves as an alternative to self-harm, and belonging to a supportive peer group can be very protective. Belonging to some *groups* seems instead to *increase* risk – for instance those attracted to the 'goth' subculture.[13] It is unclear whether this is because individuals are influenced by the beliefs of others in the group, or because membership of this sort of group appears attractive to those who are already self-harming (or both). Similar comments apply to those who prefer heavy metal music over other sorts of music.[14] Sometimes a young person feels so despairing that she doesn't expect anyone will be able to help. *Bullying* can contribute to this despair, and exacerbate low self-esteem and social isolation. Having difficulty in keeping friends, having arguments with friends, feeling lonely or breaking up from a close sexual relationship all increase the likelihood of self-harm. Exposure to self-harm in friends can be a powerful influence – the *copycat effect*.[15,16] This seems to apply especially to girls being affected by other girls cutting. An extreme form of peer influence is a *suicide pact*: it appears that mutual encouragement may at times overcome the usual inhibitions that prevent self-harm from becoming completed suicide, although such events are fortunately rare.

**BOX 27.5** Case Examples

Anthea, aged 15 years, and Stewart, aged 16 years, have been in an on-off relation-ship for two years when they each take an overdose of paracetamol at the same time. This appears to be a suicide pact. Although each is admitted to a separate ward, each is offered individual and family therapy, and they separate as a couple. They both continue to take overdoses, particularly in response to encountering each other at their educational institutions (secondary school, then college).

**BOX 27.6** Case Examples

Trevor is 15 years old when he takes his first overdose. A recent downturn in the economy has affected both his parents: his mother lost her job when a chain store stopped trading, and his father is struggling to find work as a builder. This has led to a fair amount of arguing at home. Trevor has been in an intimate relationship with a 15-year-old girl for a year, but the relationship has just broken up. She is the first person he tells about the overdose, and it becomes clear during his assessment that he wants to get back together with her.

➤ *Abuse*
  — Past *physical abuse*
  — *Sexual abuse* – Boys are more likely than girls to react to sexual abuse with self-harm.
➤ Concerns about *sexual orientation* – Young people who are concerned about being gay or bisexual, or have established that they are, are more likely to self-harm than those who are heterosexual. The self-harm may be related to homo-phobic bullying by peers or disapproval of this life choice by parents – both of which may be either real or anticipated.
➤ *Portrayals by the media* of suicide may inadvertently glorify it or encourage young people to identify with someone who has killed themselves, or learn effective methods of suicide. The impact of the media on suicidal behaviour seems to be most likely when a method of suicide is specified – especially when presented in detail – when the story is reported or portrayed dramatically and prominently, for example with photographs of the deceased or large headlines, and when suicides of celebrities are reported[17] (such as the suicide of Kurt Cobain). Young people seem to be particularly susceptible to such influences. Fictional presentations may also have an impact.[18]
➤ Debatably, exposure to some *websites* may increase the risk of self-harm. Many websites provide constructive and useful information that can aid in the under-standing of self-harm or help individuals struggling with suicidal thoughts.[19] Feedback from young people themselves about self-harm websites suggests that

they often value them as sources of empathy and understanding, as (virtual) communities, and as a way of coping with social and psychological distress.[20] Websites vary from the provision of information and leaflets to more interactive sites with chat rooms and bulletin boards that enable individuals to discuss their experiences and feelings with each other. Young people may not be able to evaluate the worth of a website, and may be unduly influenced by its appearance and layout.[21] Some easily accessible websites may glorify or encourage suicide,[22] for instance by:

— giving details of lethal methods (*recipe* sites)
— encouragement to use suicide as a problem-solving strategy
— exerting peer pressure on those who are wavering via chat rooms or bulletin boards, which may be unsupervised
— cyber-bullying, contributing to the risk of self-harm
— facilitating suicide pacts by people who have met only online.

## Significance

The seriousness of self-harm is that it predisposes to further self-harm, and in some cases to death. The repetition rate during the first year is probably at least 10%, while the lifetime risk of death is probably between 0.2% and 4.3%.[23] Factors increasing the risk of death gleaned from psychological autopsies on successful suicides include:

➤ being male
➤ being an older teenager
➤ hopelessness
➤ substance misuse
➤ multiple previous episodes, especially if some have been of a violent nature
➤ no past or current treatment or psychological support
➤ psychiatric disorder, especially depression or bipolar disorder
➤ previous psychiatric hospital admission
➤ relational problems with a partner during the past year
➤ exposure to suicidal behaviour by friends and media
➤ poor communication with parents about suicidal ideas.[24,25,26]

## WHAT MAKES YOUNG PEOPLE SELF-HARM?

Self-harm is seen as a **coping mechanism**, a way of expressing something that cannot be expressed in other ways, as described in a valuable qualitative study:

> 'There is increasing understanding and acceptance that self-harm is a response to profound emotional pain. It is a way of dealing with distress and of getting release from feelings of self-hatred, anger, sadness, depression and so on. By engaging in self-harm people may alter their state of mind so that they feel better able to cope with the other pain they are feeling.'[27]

If you ask young people who self-harm: 'What does it do for you?' or 'How does it help you?' (these are probably better questions than 'Why do you do it?'), they will often describe release of pent-up emotions, relief from unbearable feelings, or the way in which physical pain is much more bearable than their emotional pain (although it is possible that sometimes such phrases may be culled from websites). A young person who tries cutting for the first time is likely to find it a rewarding experience for these reasons, and because there is probably a physiological component: it is likely that endorphins are released in response to damaging the skin (which is very rich in nerve-endings), and that these create a kind of 'mini-high' which is desirable, repeatable and possibly to some extent addictive. For these reasons, cutting once started is moderately likely to continue.

In contrast, a young person who tries overdosing for the first time may hope the tablets will send her to sleep. Even though she may have genuinely felt that she wanted to die, she may not have thought in much depth what dying implies, particularly if the overdose was impulsive.

**Continuation** of self-harming behaviours may be due to the continual rewards experienced, such as temporary relief or release, a sense of control and the response of others.

Research has suggested some **common themes** in the purposes or reasons for self-harm,[28,29] as shown in Box 27.7. Often one young person may give several of these reasons at the same time.

**BOX 27.7** Reasons given by young people for self-harm

**Mainly inward:**
I wanted to get relief from a terrible state of mind
I wanted to escape from a situation
I wanted to get relief or release
I wanted to punish myself

**Mainly outward:**
I wanted to find out whether someone really loved me
I wanted to show how desperate I was feeling
I wanted to frighten someone
I wanted to change the behaviour of others
I wanted to get some attention

**Both inward and outward:**
I wanted to get my own back on someone/make him feel guilty
I wanted to die

Self-harming can usefully be seen as a form of communication. The communication has been described as **'a message in a bottle'**, since it is not always easy to decipher exactly what is intended (consciously or unconsciously).[30] If at least some of the communication can be heard, and if the content can be expressed in some other way, then the self-harm need not recur: teenagers are less likely to repeat the self-harm if they feel understood by those around them. Many young people say that their self-harm gets worse partly because of professional attempts to stop it without understanding and without an alternative outlet being provided for the underlying feelings.[31] In a busy Accident and Emergency department, it is all too easy to regard self-cutting as a nuisance that takes up time that could be better used for 'real' problems. Some young people who cut report that the unsympathetic and judgmental attitude of professionals to their self-harm makes their overall difficulties worse,[32] so it is important to show respect and allow time to listen to the young person's description of her predicament.[33] It is also important to appear neutral if you are shown scars or burn marks, however much revulsion you may feel. Exhibiting disgust will not endear you to the young person for whom these have become a means of emotional survival.

Thinking of the episode of self-harm as ***an attempt to communicate*** something that cannot be communicated in any other way leads to several possibilities, which may raise more questions than answers:

➤ the topic may be difficult to talk about
➤ some feelings are very difficult for anybody to describe
➤ the young person has difficulty putting feelings into words, and tends to keep things to herself
➤ the people surrounding the young person (family, friends and teachers) aren't easy to talk to.

Relatives and sometimes professionals may respond by treating the episode as trivial, *manipulative*, devious or ***attention-seeking***. These are *not* helpful ways of looking at it, even though there may be some truth in some of these views. The 'attention-seeking' hypothesis can lead to a behavioural approach to treatment that involves giving as *little attention* to the young person as possible. The danger of this is that it may lead to an escalation of self-harm (deeper cutting, more frequent overdosing) – which can achieve more attention but less understanding.

If a young person really is seeking attention, it is ***helpful sorts of attention*** that she needs, probably a great deal more of it than she has been getting. She should therefore be given the time to understand the nature of her needs. She may have a lot to cope with, and scant support to do so, although she may not necessarily tell professionals very much of her burden. A young person who self-harms may find it difficult to confide in adults, and is likely to have a coping strategy that is avoidant rather than problem-solving.[34] She is more likely to share details of her predicament if the professionals she encounters are sympathetic and supportive, and interested in understanding what might have made her self-harm. The mere fact that a young person presents for treatment, in contrast to the much higher proportion who do not, suggests a need – albeit at times ambivalent – to communicate the distress.

**BOX 27.8** Case Example: one cutter's reasons for starting (and continuing) to cut herself *(contributed anonymously with permission)*

**The first year:**
Because I felt miserable and everyone was comfortable not noticing
Because I needed something actual to confirm my misery
Because I wanted to be more special
Because it was my secret
Because I felt that no one can enter my world
Because it defined the limits of my world
Because I felt lonely
Because I hated myself
Because it was my way of educating me
Because it was my way of punishing me

**The second year:**
Because it became a habit
Because it was my way to connect my true feelings
Because it was the only way I could touch myself
Because I felt worse, but everyone kept telling me I'm making progress
Because everyone thought I was so great, except for me
Because I did what everyone wanted me to do, and it was my rebellion
Because it was the way I could destroy the doll I was for them, could kill her
Because I felt ugly and it was my punishment
Because I felt fat and it was my punishment

**The third year** (after stopping for 5 months):
Because I got hurt again
Because I suddenly understood that I hurt myself in other ways even when I thought I stopped, and I had to be punished for that
Because I felt I was contaminated
Because I had poison in me and it was the way to get it out of my system
Because I was desperate
Because it gave me the power to get out of bed and pretend
Because I felt unnecessary inside my body
Because my body brought me pain
Because I didn't care anymore
Because I wanted someone to help me

## REFERRAL

Best practice is that all children and adolescents who have taken a deliberate *overdose* should be admitted to a paediatric ward,[35,36] although local policies and age cut-offs vary. For instance, some Accident and Emergency departments send home anyone over 16 without significant medical problems, and many hospitals do not admit over-16s to a paediatric ward: they may be admitted instead to an overnight observation ward. Admission soon after an overdose is advisable for at least four reasons.

➤ The medical complications of the overdose need to be adequately managed. Intravenous infusions and the use of antidotes may be necessary, such as acetyl-cysteine for paracetamol ingestion. In some cases, prolonged observation may be needed (as in amitriptyline overdose).

➤ To enable a thorough assessment to be carried out during working hours, after the initial crisis surrounding the admission has settled.

➤ To impress upon the young person and her family the potential seriousness of her action.

➤ To create a window of opportunity for change.

It is important to remember that there need not be a correlation between *the medical and the psychological seriousness* of the episode. For instance, a girl may have taken only five paracetamol tablets, yet still genuinely wish to die (at least transiently), or be significantly depressed. Young people vary in how informed they are about the effects of too many tablets, and how many are necessary to die: many may think that the overdose will simply help them sleep for a long while, without knowing that liver damage is a potential and painful consequence.

**BOX 27.9** Case Examples

The paediatric staff of a district general hospital become concerned that there seems to be an epidemic of overdoses at the local girls' high school. They observe that many girls in years 10 and 11 have recently taken 14 or 15 paracetomol. One of them eventually admits that her friend told her: 'You have to take at least 16 to kill yourself', so she stopped short of taking the whole packet of 16.

This is discussed at the weekly ward psychosocial discussion meeting. It is calculated that the reason there seem to be more admissions from that school than the local boys' and mixed schools is simply because there are so many more girls at the school. It is also agreed that there does seem to be a significant copycat element to the recent sequence of admissions.

The lead paediatrician contacts the head teacher of the girls' high school to discuss whether it would be worth giving some tuition to all pupils in year 10 and 11 about the potential dangers of paracetomol. The head teacher agrees to discuss this idea with the school educational psychologist and the governors. The outcome of this is that the school agrees to adopt guidelines on the management of self-harm within schools[37,38] and to introduce tuition in problem-solving skills to Personal, Health and Social Education lessons – but there is no tuition about the dangers of paracetomol.

**TABLE 27.1** When, and when not, to refer self-cutting

| Does not need referral | Referral should be discussed |
| --- | --- |
| Superficial cutting, leading to little bleeding, and scars that heal quickly | Deep scars, some needing stitching |
| Nothing to indicate abuse | A known history of sexual abuse or rape, or promiscuous sexual activity |
| No other self-harm | Association with overdosing |
| No history of bingeing, vomiting or distorted body image | Association with an eating disorder |
| A sensible attitude to experimentation with drugs and alcohol | Use of drugs or alcohol that is potentially dangerous |
| Mood changes are transient | Persistent depression or anxiety |

In reality, as Figure 27.1 shows, young people who self-harm *mostly do not seek any professional input*, and if they do pluck up the courage to talk to a professional, may not want to be passed on to another. For an adolescent who discloses an overdose long after it has happened, referral to a hospital paediatric ward is likely to be pointless, but the young person should still be advised to seek an appointment with her GP for review and assessment. A referral to a specialised CAMHS service would be indicated if there are persisting mental health issues such as depression.

Young people who *cut* themselves or self-injure in other minor ways should in general not be referred. However, some of them may have associated problems that deserve referral in their own right, as summarised in Table 27.1. Those whose cuts are deep enough may need some treatment in an Accident and Emergency department. Some may be cutting because of past sexual abuse, and may benefit from some counselling about this, although many do not want this, or are not yet ready for it – which should be respected. Ongoing sexual abuse probably needs to be reported to the local social services duty office if this has not happened already (an exception to this would be an over-16 year old who refuses to give permission for you to report her abuse to the authorities: you must override this if you believe a younger child is seriously at risk). (*See* Chapter 12 on Child Abuse and Safeguarding.) Other psychiatric disorders may need treatment in their own right, such as eating disorders, substance misuse, depression or emerging borderline personality disorder.

A comment on *confidentiality* may be relevant here (*see also* Chapter 43: Consent, Competence, Capacity and Confidentiality). A young person may not want you to tell her parents about her self-harm. Such a desire for secrecy should be respected unless there is a danger of death. So in general, simple cutting does not justify a breach of confidentiality. An overdose however may, especially if you consider the young person's life may be at risk. If you are going to tell her parents, you must tell her first, and explain to her why you think this is necessary, in terms of her parents needing to know before she dies rather than after, and your duty to them as well as to her. If you put enough effort into explaining this, she is likely to accept the need for a parent to be told of the danger she is in. If life seems endangered, similar comments apply to the need for referral to another professional or team.

**BOX 27.10** Case Example

Cynthia, a depressed but high-achieving 16-year-old girl, is attending regular appointments with her CAMHS worker following a paracetomol overdose that was assessed as having high suicidal intent. Cynthia tells her counsellor that she knows where her father keeps the key to his gun cabinet (the counsellor had no idea there were any guns in the household). Cynthia reveals that she has been dwelling for some time on a plan to remove one of her father's shotguns and take it up to the top of the nearest hill on order to shoot herself.

The counsellor does not conceal that she is rather taken aback by this, and very concerned. She explains that this is not the sort of information that she can keep to herself: it is essential that Cynthia's parents are informed. Cynthia accepts this, and agrees to allow the counsellor to tell her father what she has said (but the counsellor would have had to tell him even without Cynthia's consent). He is suitably concerned, and agrees to find a more secure place for the gun cabinet key.

Cynthia subsequently accepts further appointments, continuing to see her counsellor. She recovers from her depression, gets excellent A-level grades, and attends a prestigious university.

## ASSESSMENT

Referral may be dictated by the nature of the self-harm, such as a recent overdose, in which case a detailed prior assessment may be superfluous. If referral is not immediately indicated, an assessment should aim to develop some understanding of the **context and intent** of the self-harm. Incorporating therapeutic elements into the assessment may improve engagement and attendance at any follow-up appointments.[39] The order of the questions should go from most gentle and open to most searching and closed. For convenience, examples of questions that could be used are here grouped in three categories: one general and one each relating to the two main types of self-harm – but they should not necessarily be asked in this order. Factual details about the recent episode and any previous self-harm should be gathered first. It should be noted that asking about suicide does not make it more likely to occur.

Questions relating to **self-harm in general** may include the following.

➤ Has anything happened recently to bother you? (This is an open question that could lead on to further enquiries about life events.)

➤ How are school/family life/friendships? (The exact wording will vary.)

➤ Who is living at home? Who do you get on best with? Who do you find it most difficult to get on with?

➤ Has anyone you know (or know of) committed suicide or self-harmed?

➤ How long did you plan harming yourself? Or was it done just on impulse? (People may die from impulsive self-harm, particularly hanging, but in general it is of lower risk than a long-intended and carefully planned piece of self-destruction.)

➤ How happy are you on a scale of 1–10, with 10 being the happiest you could be and zero being the saddest you could be? Now? At the time of the self-harm?

➤ There should usually be some enquiry about abuse, but not as an opening question, and only if you feel you have established sufficient rapport for such a question to be acceptable. It should be open enough to include a variety of forms of abuse, but specific enough to make it clear what you mean. 'Has anyone ever done anything to you that you think they shouldn't have?' may be too vague. Alternatives include: 'Some teenagers who self-harm have been bullied or physically abused or sexually abused or raped. Has any of these happened to you?' or 'The sort of feelings that lead to self-harm sometimes arise from something traumatic in the past that is very unpleasant to remember. Do you think that might apply to you?' (This allows the possibility of acknowledging past abuse without talking about any details.)

➤ What information have you found out about self-harm?

➤ What goes through your mind as you harm yourself? (This is sometimes too difficult to answer.)

After an **overdose**, some suggested questions include the following.

➤ Did you try to avoid being found out? (A young person who ensures she is alone in the house before taking an overdose is likely to be more at risk of completed suicide than one who ensures there is someone there.)

➤ What persuaded you to tell someone? (Often this is the onset of physical symptoms such as vomiting or stomach cramps, which the young person may find scary.)

➤ When did you tell someone? (The delay until someone was told is one among several indicators of suicidal intent.)

➤ Did you write a suicide note or blog? (Another indicator of increased suicidal risk.)

➤ Did you think it would kill you?
  – If yes, try to explore what dying means to the young person: is it perhaps a metaphor for escaping from an unbearable situation or avoiding unbearable feelings? Is it the pain that needs to be killed? *See* Box 27.7.
  – If no, explore what she *did* expect. A common answer can be: 'I wanted to go to sleep (for a long time).' If so, what makes being awake so undesirable?

➤ Do you want to die now (still)? (The answer is usually 'No' after an overdose, which generally leads to a rebound in mood: a 'Yes' answer is worrying.)

A brief summary of the salient questions after an overdose is contained in the PATHOS questionnaire, shown in Box 27.5, which gives a score out of five as a rough guide to the level of risk: higher scores correlate with suicidal intent and depression.[40]

**BOX 27.11** The PATHOS Questionnaire

| | |
|---|---|
| 'Have you had **Problems** for longer than one month?' | [P] |
| 'Were you **Alone** in the house when you overdosed?' | [A] |
| 'Did you plan the overdose for more than **Three** hours?' | [T] |
| 'Are you feeling **Hopeless** about the future – that things won't get much better?' | [HO] |
| 'Were you feeling **Sad** for most of the time before the overdose?' | [S] |
| Score one point for each item present, and total out of five. | |

A more detailed summary that allows a score of potential suicide risk, the Pierce Suicide Intent Scale, is shown in Table 27.2. The answers should emerge from the assessment indicated above.

As **cutting** is likely to be repeated, questions about the latest episode may or may not be so useful. Questions specific to cutting can include the following.

➤ What do you use?
➤ What part of the body do you mainly cut?
➤ Do you tell anyone about it?
➤ Does it make you feel better?
➤ If so, how do you think it does this?
➤ What do you feel immediately after you have cut?
➤ Have you tried any alternatives to cutting?

## MANAGEMENT AND PREVENTION

### Preventive opportunities

*Primary prevention* of youth suicide or self-harm involves targeting the whole population. Examples include the following:

➤ the restriction of opportunities for suicide such as the removal of carbon monoxide from domestic gas and the restriction of packet sizes for painkillers[41]
➤ modifying factors that might predispose young people to suicidal phenomena, such as by changing attitudes or improving coping skills
➤ media adherence to guidelines about the portrayal of suicide
➤ regulation of websites giving information about self-harm or support to self-harmers.

*Secondary prevention* involves identifying those young people who may be at risk of self-harm or suicide and targeting them for professional help.

*Tertiary prevention* involves trying to prevent further self-harm after it has already begun. One reason for the importance of admission after the first overdose is that it creates an opportunity for doing this properly. Families are more likely to change when anxiety levels are high rather than a few days or weeks later, and management is more likely to be successful when the young person first presents than when the behaviour becomes a chronic pattern.

Suggestions for primary prevention strategies in schools are given below.

**TABLE 27.2** The Pierce Suicide Intent Scale

| | **Circumstances and actions** | | |
|---|---|---|---|
| 1 | Isolation | 0 | Somebody present |
| | | 1 | Somebody nearby or in contact, e.g. by phone |
| | | 2 | No one nearby or in contact |
| 2 | Timing | 0 | Timed so that intervention is probable |
| | | 1 | Timed so that intervention is not likely |
| | | 2 | Timed so that intervention is highly unlikely |
| 3 | Precautions against | 0 | No precautions |
| | discovery and/or intervention | 1 | Passive precautions, e.g. avoiding others but doing nothing to prevent intervention (alone in room, door unlocked) |
| | | 2 | Active precautions such as locking doors |
| 4 | Action to gain help during or | 0 | Notified potential helper regarding attempt |
| | after the attempt | 1 | Contacted but did not specifically notify potential helper regarding the attempt |
| | | 2 | Did not contact or notify potential helper |
| 5 | Final acts in anticipation of | 0 | None |
| | death | 1 | Partial preparation or ideation |
| | | 2 | Definite plans made |
| 6 | Suicide note | 0 | Absence of note |
| | | 1 | Note written but torn up |
| | | 2 | Presence of note |
| | **Self-report** | | |
| 1 | Patient's statement of | 0 | Thought what s/he had done would not kill him/her |
| | lethality | 1 | Unsure whether what s/he had done would kill him/her |
| | | 2 | Believed what s/he had done would kill him/her |
| 2 | Stated intent | 0 | Did not want to die |
| | | 1 | Uncertain or did not care if s/he lived or died |
| | | 2 | Did want to die |
| 3 | Premeditation | 0 | Impulsive, no premeditation |
| | | 1 | Considered act for less than one hour |
| | | 2 | Considered act for less than one day |
| | | 3 | Considered act for more than one day |
| 4 | Reaction to the act | 0 | Patient glad s/he has recovered |
| | | 1 | Patient is uncertain whether s/he is sorry |
| | | 2 | Patient is sorry s/he has recovered |
| | **Risk** | | |
| 1 | Predictable outcome in terms | 0 | Survival certain |
| | of lethality of patient's act | 1 | Death unlikely |
| | and circumstances known to | 2 | Death likely or certain |
| | him/her | | |
| 2 | Would death have occurred | 0 | No |
| | without medical treatment ? | 1 | Uncertain |
| | | 2 | Yes |

TOTAL SCORE =

(Low intent = 0–3          Medium intent = 4–10          High intent = 11–21)

### Communication and support

Young people – and some parents – may obtain information and/or support from some of the websites listed below under Resources. Although most young people seem to value such websites,[42] there are risks, as specified above. Parental attempts to filter the websites their children can access are variable and may need more government support.[43,44] The Australian government banned pro-suicide websites in 2006, but website optimisation strategies may have more impact – by preferentially directing suicidal young people to helpful rather than potentially harmful sites.[45]

The single most helpful thing a professional can do after an act of self-harm is to **encourage communication** between the adolescent in crisis and important others around her. These may include family, boyfriend, other friends and schoolteachers. She may need help to say what is bothering her. It can be a big relief for the young person to have her hitherto secretive behaviour accepted, making it a little easier to talk about. In some cases, it is impossible to decipher the message within the bottle, but this does not necessarily matter, providing channels of communication become more available. Other sources of support may be necessary, such as a counsellor at school or in a voluntary organisation, a crisis helpline, or websites such as those listed below as resources. If you can find out which websites the young person is using, then you can check them out or ask her parents to check that they are supportive rather than liable to encourage suicide.

With parents who are angry or ashamed about their daughter's action, it is important to **reframe these emotions** as evidence of concern, in other words construing these emotions in a positive light. You could say, for instance, (to the adolescent in her parents' presence): 'It is clear that your parents are very worried about you. They are quite right to be concerned. It shows how much they care about you.' Try to reinforce the concern element of the parents' feelings – rather than the blame element.

An **interview with the adolescent on her own** is essential, to explore the meaning of the episode and the degree of suicidal intent (of which parents are usually unaware). With her permission, a version of this can be told to the family. This is in many cases sufficient to enable the family to understand the message in the bottle. It may be necessary at times to talk to other agencies, such as the school in cases of academic pressure or bullying, or social services in cases of abuse.

In the case of self-cutting, the upset and shame arising from unsightly scars may need to be acknowledged. Negative connotations can be reduced by **informing the young person and her parents that cutting is**:

➤ **common** – probably much commoner than they think
➤ **difficult to stop**, because the physiological effects give so much relief and release
➤ **seldom dangerous** – providing the cutting remains superficial
➤ potentially **protective**, by stopping the young person from doing something worse; cutting can be a way of dealing with feelings that would otherwise lead to an overdose[46]

➤ an effective and relatively safe way for the young person to *express feelings* – a bit like slamming doors or shouting.

This may result in a more permissive attitude by parents towards cutting, which in turn may enable the young person to be more open about it.

**BOX 27.12** Case Example

At the age of 15 years, Emma is brought by her friends to the drop-in clinic run by the community school nurse at her school. They are concerned that she has been cutting herself and has talked to them about her cutting being a good way of managing stress. Emma agreed to meet individually with the school nurse and talk through some of the issues for her.

Emma informs the school nurse that she has recently split up with her boyfriend and has been getting very distressed at seeing him going out with another girl in her class. She has developed the habit of cutting her arms in the evenings while alone in her bedroom and listening to her favourite music. She has found that the cutting relieves her tension and makes her feel better. She denies any suicidal thoughts. She has not told her mother what she is doing, but she thinks her mother might have an idea, since she walked into Emma's bedroom on one occasion when Emma was cleaning up after a cutting episode.

Emma is keen to talk more about her feelings. The school nurse tells Emma that they can meet on a regular basis if Emma wishes. In view of the frequency of the cutting, she asks Emma's permission to tell her mother about the situation. Although tearful about this, Emma reluctantly agrees to the school nurse telephoning Emma's mother.

The school nurse calls Emma's mother to explain her concerns and to inform her that Emma has agreed to come to the drop-in clinic regularly. The school nurse also consults with the primary mental health worker and they discuss strategies that the school nurse can use for helping Emma to manage her self-harm. They also discuss the level of risk, and whether there is anything further they need to do about this. They agree that the school nurse will contact the primary mental health worker again if Emma appears to be getting depressed or suicidal or expanding her repertoire of self-harm.

Emma attends the drop-in clinic weekly. She informs the school nurse that she has had a long talk with her mother, prompted by the surprise phone call. Emma has eventually been able to agree with her mother that she will no longer shut herself up in her room on her own in the evenings, when her cutting is most likely to occur, but will distract herself by doing something with other family members. She has also started using a diary to write down her feelings.

After several more weeks of coming to the drop-in clinic, Emma reports that her cutting seems to feel less necessary; she explains that she thinks she is now managing her feelings in other ways. Soon after this, she meets a new boyfriend and stops attending the drop-in clinic. Reports to the school nurse from teachers give no cause for concern, so no further action is taken.

**ALTERNATIVES TO CUTTING**[47,48]

These are worth discussing with any young person who is cutting, although many will report back that no other activity quite 'does it' for them in the way that cutting does. **Alternative ways of discharging unpleasant emotions** include the following:

➤ having a rubber band around a forearm and twanging it
➤ clenching ice cubes in a hand until they melt
➤ hitting a pillow or soft object that won't mind being hit
➤ going into a field or cellar and screaming
➤ writing a letter expressing feelings – which need not be sent
➤ any form of aerobic exercise, the more strenuous the better
➤ martial arts.

Some of these can work by distraction. Other **distraction techniques** include the following:

➤ keeping a diary or blog
➤ writing poetry
➤ playing or composing music
➤ drawing or painting
➤ do-it-yourself or carpentry
➤ taking a pet dog for a walk
➤ talking to friends or family
➤ communicating with others electronically, for instance through a messenger service or on a social networking site such as 'Facebook'[49]
➤ doing something sociable, such as going to the cinema with friends
➤ reading a book
➤ listening to loud music.

There are also ways of **self-soothing**, which may help some young people:

➤ stroking a pet such as a cat or guinea pig
➤ having a bubble bath
➤ listening to soothing music
➤ practising breathing and relaxation techniques
➤ anaerobic exercise such as yoga
➤ mindfulness techniques such as:
   — going to a park and looking at the trees and flowers and birds
   — walking in a quiet place and listening to the surrounding sounds
   — staying with an emerging emotion rather than trying to avoid it or suppress it (young people who self-harm may find this particularly difficult)
   — sitting still and focusing on the in-breath and out-breath (or other forms of meditation).

**MEASURES IN SCHOOLS**[50]

Preventive measures in schools have received increasing attention: they may involve teachers, pupils and others.[51,52] Elements of successful *school intervention programmes* include *specific* and *universal* interventions. Interventions specific to self-harm, or factors leading to self-harm such as depression, have not been proven to be worth their cost;[53] universal interventions such as those affecting **the climate of the school** are generally thought to be more effective (*see also* Chapter 6 on Resilience and Risk).[54,55] Schools that encourage resilience and increase mental health and well-being in general seem to be those that:

➤ promote a **focus on learning** in an organised and supportive way (for instance cultivating an ethos of academic achievement and positive feedback from teachers about work done)

➤ encourage pupil **autonomy** (for instance the pursuit of personal interests and the allowance of self-expression – saying what you think)

➤ encourage **harmony** and decrease conflict between pupils and between teachers and pupils (for instance reducing fighting and bullying between pupils and reducing authoritarian components of discipline such as teachers shouting at pupils)

➤ maintain professional **boundaries** between teachers and pupils (for instance each treating the other with respect and teachers keeping their personal lives out of the classroom).

Interventions specific to self-harm *may* also be helpful, but need to be in place for extended periods of time (at least a school year) and should involve everyone associated with the school (staff, pupils, parents, visiting professionals and governors), so they may be too costly to be realistic. One such programme, developed in Pennsylvania, has been piloted in three parts of the UK and evaluated by the London School of Economics.[56] To be successful, it seems that such interventions need to include at least some of the following components.

➤ Teaching and other school staff need to be informed about how to accept self-harm in a non-judgmental way and listen to the young person's concerns, rather than immediately passing the problem onto someone else, or worse still, asking the young person to leave the school! Support for teachers may be provided by a school counsellor or community school nurse.

➤ Lessons (probably in Personal, Health and Social Education) can include teaching on:

— the development of suicidality from thoughts about suicide to attempts to completion

— the possible biopsychosocial factors leading to self-harm, depression or suicide

— removing the stigma about mental health difficulties and seeking help for them – this is not specific to self-harm[57]

— problem-solving skills involving case vignettes

— strategies for coping with stressful situations

— the identification of specific verbal and behavioural warning signs in others (and oneself)

— giving information regarding available school-based and community-based resources for help.

➤ This teaching can form the basis for peer intervention: all pupils can be taught how to detect the signs of possible impending depression or suicide in their friends and acquaintances, and how to offer their own support or connect the other young person with support from professionals. Peer responses that can be taught include:
  — building up the conditions for communication
  — active listening – asking questions and showing concern
  — encouraging help-seeking behaviour
  — using a guideline such as in Box 27.13.

**BOX 27.13** My friend has a problem: how can I help?

You can help a lot by just being there and listening.
If you feel that is not enough, encourage your friend to seek help from an adult. This could be a teacher, a counsellor, a school nurse or a parent.
You can offer to go with your friend.
If you are worried enough, you may have to tell an adult yourself, but you should tell your friend you are going to do this.
You may feel stirred up by all this, or your friend may feel angry with you – so make sure you have some adult support for yourself.

**BOX 27.14** Some Alarm Bells in relation to self-harm

A suicide note, blog or e-mail
Attempts to avoid detection
Availability of dangerous things in cupboards, such as large amounts of aspirin or paracetomol, or an adult's tricyclic antidepressants
Hopelessness
Substance misuse
Poor lines of communication with friends and family
Influences from acquaintances or the media

**BOX 27.15** Practice Points for self-harm

Overnight hospital admission is recommended immediately after any overdose for all under-18s.
  Other young people with self-harm may be managed in the community, but specialist referral will be necessary if suicidal risk is assessed as high or there are serious mental health issues such as depression.

All self-harmers should be treated with respect and given time and attention. Cutting should be regarded as a solution as well as a problem.

Assessment should be based on an understanding of how self-harm:

- functions as a coping strategy
- regulates emotions
- may be communicating something, even if it is not clear what.

Management may include:

- enhancing communication between the young person and others (family members and friends)
- encouraging a permissive attitude to cutting
- introducing alternatives to self-harm.

## RESOURCES

### *Websites specifically relating to self-harm or suicidality*

- Papyrus has a good information leaflet for parents on Internet safety and runs a helpline for young people called HOPELineUK on 0800 0684141 for practical advice on suicide prevention.
- www.papyrus-uk.org
- www.papyrus-uk.org/pdf/ACTion.pdf
- Samaritans: www.samaritans.org
- MIND: www.mind.org.uk/help/diagnoses_and_conditions/about_self-harm_a_guide_for_young_people
- An information leaflet from the Royal College of Psychiatrists: www.rcpsych.ac.uk/mentalhealthinfo/problems/depression/self-harm.aspx

### More general websites:

- Childline has a helpline on 0800 1111.
  www.childline.org.uk
- Young Minds: www.youngminds.org.uk
- Teenage Health Freak: www.teenagehealthfreak.org
- Ask Dr Ann: www.teenagehealthfreak.org/askdrann

## REFERENCES

1 National Institute for Health and Clinical Excellence. *Self-harm: the short-term physical and psychological management and secondary prevention of self-harm in primary and secondary care.* London: NICE; 2004. Available at: www.nice.org.uk/CG016 (accessed 31 March 2011)
2 Madge N, Hewitt A, Hawton K, *et al.* Deliberate self-harm within an international community sample of young people: comparative findings from the Child & Adolescent Self-harm in Europe (CASE) Study. *J Child Psychol Psychiatry.* 2008; **49**(6): 667–77.
3 Rodham K, Hawton K, Evans E. Reasons for deliberate self-harm: comparison of self-poisoners and self-cutters in a community sample of adolescents. *J Am Acad Child Adolesc Psychiatry.* 2004; **43**(1): 80–7.

4 Runeson B, Tidemalm D, Dahlin M, *et al.* Method of attempted suicide as predictor of subsequent successful suicide: national long term cohort study. *BMJ.* 2010; **341**: 186.

5 Hawton K, Rodham K, Evans E. *By Their Own Young Hand: deliberate self-harm and suicidal ideas in adolescents.* London: Jessica Kingsley Publishers; 2006.

6 Yip K. A multi-dimensional perspective of adolescents' self-cutting. *Child and Adolescent Mental Health.* 2005; **10**(2): 80–6.

7 Sarkar M, Byrne P, Power L. Are suicidal phenomena in children different to suicidal phenomena in adolescents? A six-year review. *Child and Adolescent Mental Health.* 2010; **15**(4): 197–203.

8 Hawton, 2006, op. cit.

9 Hawton, 2006, op. cit. p. 82.

10 de Leo D, Heller T. Social modeling in the transmission of suicidality. *Crisis.* 2008; **29**(1): 11–19.

11 Speckens AE, Hawton K. Social problem solving in adolescents with suicidal behavior: a systematic review. *Suicide and Life-Threatening Behavior.* 2005; **35**(4): 365–87.

12 Evans E, Hawton K, Rodham K. In what ways are adolescents who engage in self-harm or experience thoughts of self-harm different in terms of help-seeking, communication and coping strategies? *Journal of Adolescence.* 2005; **28**(4): 573–87.

13 Young R, Sweeting H, West P. Prevalence of deliberate self harm and attempted suicide within contemporary Goth youth subculture: longitudinal cohort study. *BMJ.* 2006; **332**(7549): 1058–61.

14 Hawton, 2006, op. cit.

15 de Leo, op. cit.

16 Ho T, Leung P, Hung S, *et al.* The Mental Health of the Peers of Suicide Completers and Attempters. *Journal of Child Psychology and Psychiatry.* 2000; **41**(3): 301–8.

17 Hawton K, Williams K. Influences of the media on suicide. *BMJ.* 2002; **325**(7377): 1374–5.

18 Hawton K, Simkin S, Deeks JJ, *et al.* Effects of a drug overdose in a television drama on presentations to hospital for self poisoning: time series and questionnaire study. *BMJ.* 1999; **318**(7189): 972–7.

19 Hawton, 2006, op. cit.

20 Baker D, Fortune S. Understanding self-harm and suicide websites: a qualitative interview study of young adult website users. *Crisis.* 2008; **29**(3): 118–22.

21 Hawton, 2006, op. cit.

22 Biddle L, Donovan J, Hawton K, *et al.* Suicide and the Internet. *BMJ.* 2008; **336**(7648): 800–2.

23 Hawton K, James A. Suicide and deliberate self harm in young people. *BMJ.* 2005; **330**(7496): 891–4.

24 Hawton, 2005, op. cit.

25 Portzky G, Audenaert K, van Heeringen K. Psychosocial and psychiatric factors associated with adolescent suicide: a case control psychological autopsy study. *Journal of Adolescence.* 2009; **32**: 849–62.

26 Hawton, 2006, op. cit.

27 Mental Health Foundation. *Truth Hurts – Report of the National Enquiry into Self-Harm among Young People.* London: Mental Health Foundation; 2006.

28 Scoliers G, Portzky G, Madge N, *et al.* Reasons for adolescent deliberate self-harm: a cry of pain and/or a cry for help? Findings from the child and adolescent self-harm in Europe (CASE) study. *Soc Psychiatry Psychiatr Epidemiol.* 2009; **44**(8): 601–7.

29 Hawton, 2006, op. cit.

30 Kingsbury S. Parasuicide in adolescence: a message in a bottle. *ACPP Rev Newsletter*. 1993; **15**: 253–9.

31 Spandler H, Warner S. *Beyond Fear and Control: working with young people who self-harm*. Ross-on-Wye: PCCS Books; 2007.

32 Mental Health Foundation, op. cit.

33 National Institute for Health and Clinical Excellence, op. cit.

34 Evans, 2005, op. cit.

35 National Institute for Health and Clinical Excellence, op. cit.

36 Department of Health. *National Service Framework for children, young people and maternity services*. London: Department of Health; 2004.

37 Hawton, 2006, op. cit.

38 Oxfordshire Adolescent Self Harm Forum. *Self Harm: guidelines for staff within school and residential settings*. Oxford: Oxfordshire Adolescent Self Harm Forum; 2006. Available for £5 from Dr Anne Stewart, Boundary Brook House, Churchill Drive, Headington, Oxford OX3 7LQ.

39 Ougrin D, Zundel T, Ng A, *et al.* Trial of Therapeutic Assessment in London: randomised controlled trial of Therapeutic Assessment versus standard psychosocial self-harm assessment in adolescents presenting with self-harm. *Arch Dis Child*. 2011 Feb; **96**(2): 148–53.

40 Kingsbury S. PATHOS: a screening instrument for adolescent overdose: a research note. *Journal of Child Psychology and Psychiatry*. 1996; **37**(5): 609–11.

41 Hawton K, Simkin S, Deeks JJ, *et al.* UK legislation on analgesic packs: before and after study of long term effect on poisonings. *BMJ*. 2004; **329**(7474): 1076–9.

42 Baker, op. cit.

43 Coombes R. Safety Nets. *BMJ*. 2008; **336**(7648): 803.

44 Byron T. *Safer Children in a Digital World: report of the Byron Review*. London: Department for Children, Schools and Families and Department for Culture, Media and Sport; 2008. Available at: www.dcsf.gov.uk/byronreview (accessed 31 March 2011).

45 Biddle, op. cit.

46 Mental Health Foundation, op. cit.

47 Oxfordshire Adolescent Self Harm Forum, op. cit.

48 Hawton, 2006, op. cit.

49 www.facebook.com

50 This section has benefited from advice given by Dr Chrissy Boardman, Associate Specialist Child Psychiatrist, Dorset Healthcare Foundation Trust.

51 Hawton, 2006, op. cit.

52 Portzky G, van Heeringen K. Suicide prevention in adolescents: a controlled study of the effectiveness of a school-based psycho-educational program. *J Child Psychol Psychiatry*. 2006; **47**(9): 910–18.

53 Spence S, Shortt A. Research review: can we justify the widespread dissemination of universal school based interventions for the prevention of depression among children and adolescents? *J Child Psychol Psychiatry*. 2007; **48**(6): 526–42.

54 Kasen S, Cohen P, Chen H, *et al.* School climate and continuity of adolescent personality disorder symptoms. *J Child Psychol Psychiatry*. 2009; **50**(12): 1504–12.

55 Rutter M, Maughan B. *Fifteen Thousand Hours: secondary schools and their effects on children*. 2nd ed. London: Sage; 1994.

56 www.ppc.sas.upenn.edu/prpsum.htm

57 Pinfold V, Toulmin HR, Thornicroft G, *et al.* Reducing psychiatric stigma and discrimination: evaluation of educational interventions in UK secondary schools. *British Journal of Psychiatry.* 2003; **182**: 342–6.

# CHAPTER 28

# Eating disorders

## INTRODUCTION
### Overview
Children and adolescents can have a range of difficulties with eating. Child mental health professionals are often asked about:
➤ selective eating in younger children, which is common and generally harmless
➤ restrictive eating in adolescents, which is rare but potentially life-threatening
➤ excessive eating, which is common and can have significant health implications when extreme.

Although we give definitions in the next section which make it sound as if each eating disorder is different from the others, there is in reality a great deal of overlap. For instance: children who present with food faddiness may have mothers with eating disorder traits;[1] bulimia nervosa may co-exist either with obesity or with severe malnourishment; an adolescent who recovers from anorexia nervosa may subsequently develop bulimia nervosa; and, more generally, there is movement in every possible direction between the three main categories of anorexia, bulimia and atypical eating disorders.[2] In addition, many young people may have features of one or more of these conditions but not fit into a strict diagnosis.

Before we define the different presenting patterns, an assessment tool needs to be introduced that is particularly useful in the assessment of eating disorders, which we will use in the Case Examples: ***body mass index*** (BMI). This is a measure of nutritional status that compares weight to height: the formula is the weight in kilograms divided by the square of the height in metres (on a calculator, you can divide the weight by the height, and then by the height again). It supplements the ordinary growth chart that plots weight and height. Because of the variation of body mass index with age, it requires its own additional chart. For those who do not have ready access to such charts, a table summarising the most important lower limits is given as an appendix to this chapter (Table 28.1).

### Common definitions
***Selective eating/meal refusal/food faddiness*** – This is very common in preschool children, who often refuse to eat *when* carers want or *what* carers want. Although

**TABLE 28.1** Lower limits for body mass index in girls: second and ninth centiles

| Age in years | Second centile for BMI | Ninth centile for BMI |
| --- | --- | --- |
| 18 | 18.1 | 16.9 |
| 17 | 17.8 | 15.7 |
| 16 | 17.5 | 16.3 |
| 15 | 17.0 | 15.9 |
| 14 | 16.5 | 15.5 |
| 13 | 16.0 | 15.0 |
| 12 | 15.4 | 14.4 |
| 11 | 14.9 | 13.9 |
| 10 | 14.5 | 13.5 |
| 9 | 14.1 | 13.2 |
| 8 | 13.9 | 13.0 |
| 7 | 13.7 | 12.9 |
| 6 | 13.6 | 12.9 |
| 5 | 13.8 | 13.0 |

it may seem superficially similar to other oppositional behaviours, its origins may be different. The authors have experience of children who seem to have inherited heightened taste sensitivity from a parent. Some faddy children have parents whose anxiety about eating or selectivity in relation to food may interfere with the introduction to the child of new foods. Other children have experienced a choking episode or had problems as babies with gastro-oesophageal reflux: each of these experiences can make food aversive in general, or at least some foods aversive. For many children, food refusal may be the way in which the child communicates that something is either physically or emotionally not quite right.

If the limitation of food intake is severe, persistent or leads to weight loss or failure to gain weight, it is worth considering whether there is a developmental problem, such as poor coordination between the different movements required for eating (oral motor dysfunction); persisting gastro-oesophageal reflux; or autistic spectrum disorder, which may lead to the selection of food by texture, taste, brand, presentation or appearance.[3]

**BOX 28.1** Case Example

A nine-year-old boy eats nothing but yeast extract (Marmite), bread, margarine and milk. A full dietary assessment reveals that his dietary intake is adequate in quality and quantity, and his growth chart is satisfactory. The paediatric dietician agrees with his mother that no further management is needed.

*Obesity* – This is increasingly common. It can be defined in various ways, but in general is characterised by excessive weight for age and height, or excessive body mass index for age. The prevalence varies with the definition used, and between countries. Genetic factors probably play at least as important a part as cultural and other environmental factors (such as advertising). There is evidence of continuity between childhood and adult obesity, but this is not inevitable. Some overweight children become thinner during the adolescent growth spurt, particularly if they are genetically programmed to be tall adults.

*Anorexia nervosa* – The core beliefs driving this condition are *over-concern about weight and shape* and *determined avoidance of food* or overall food restriction: thinness is seen as *good* and fattening food as *bad*. In addition to limiting calorie intake, *compensatory behaviours* often occur, such as vomiting, excessive exercise or laxative abuse (purging). There is generally no loss of appetite – so in a sense 'anorexia' is a misnomer (*an* means without and *orexis* means appetite).

Cut-off numbers to start worrying are a weight below 85% of what would be expected for height, a body mass index below the ninth centile, or a rate of weight loss of more than 0.5 kg per week. The trend in weight loss may be more clinically alarming than the absolute weight: a 15-year-old girl of normal weight who has been losing weight rapidly may be of more concern than another who has been significantly underweight for some time, but is maintaining this weight. If poor weight gain persists for a significant period, then *stunting* occurs (slower growth in height), making it more difficult to interpret the growth chart – unless past measurements of height are available. In females, cessation of periods after they have started (secondary amenorrhoea) can be a useful symptom with which to engage an adolescent girl, who may be prepared to share your concern that her body is not functioning as it should, while not accepting that she is underweight. The oral contraceptive pill may cause confusion, however, as bleeding may occur during the gap in each pill cycle when it would not occur without the pill.

Anorexia nervosa mostly occurs soon after the onset of puberty: the peak incidence is around 15–18 years.[4] It is much commoner in girls than boys, with a ratio of about 10 : 1, although there may be a higher ratio of boys in prepubertal children,[5] sometimes associated with autistic traits.[6] Prepubertal onset occurs rarely, but can then permanently impair growth, bone mineralization and ovarian development. Strictly defined anorexia nervosa is a rare condition: prevalence estimates vary from about one per 100 000 for under-13s[7] to about 0.7% for teenage girls.[8] Lesser degrees or variants of the condition are commoner (*see* atypical eating disorders below), and it is important for universal and Tier 1 services to be aware of when it is possible to prevent anorexic behaviours and beliefs becoming worse, and when things have got so bad that referral is necessary (*see* below under management and referral).

**BOX 28.2** Case Example

Alisha is 13 years old when she decides she is fat, particularly in her legs, and refuses to eat or drink. Her mother asks the general practitioner for help. He notes that she does not seem dehydrated, and Alisha admits she does drink some water when she is really thirsty. She has lost weight, but there are no recent past measurements, so it is unclear how much. Her periods have not yet started. She is now on the 50th centile for height and the 25th for weight, with a body mass index of 15.1, on the second centile. After referral to a Tier 3 service, she is diagnosed with anorexia nervosa.

Alisha's mother is on her own at home with little support from the extended family or from Alisha's father, who visits occasionally. The team at the specialist CAMHS service recommend immediate admission to a paediatric ward for observation and reestablishment of a normal diet. Alisha and her mother very much do *not* want this, so it is agreed that she will go home with intensive support from the team including frequent home visits. Reluctantly, so as not to be admitted to hospital, Alisha starts eating and drinking more, but she still complains of how fat her legs look.

*Bulimia nervosa* is characterised by recurrent bingeing and vomiting. *Binges* consist of the consumption of a large amount of food in a short time, accompanied by a sense of lack of control. Often the young person compulsively chooses calorie-rich food that rapidly leads to a feeling of fullness. Binges are often followed by self-induced *vomiting*. Other *compensatory behaviours* as in anorexia nervosa may also occur, such as laxative abuse, exercise or fasting. Self-evaluation tends to be unduly influenced by body weight and shape. Typically, a young person develops a characteristic cyclical pattern of missing meals in the early part of the day with bingeing and vomiting in the evening.[9] The next day, guilt leads to renewed efforts to cut back on eating, with maintenance of the cycle. The classic bulimic strikes a balance between calorie input and compensation, and so is of roughly normal weight – although she invariably thinks she is fat. Some may be underweight, and may overlap in clinical features with anorexia nervosa. Others may be overweight.

Bulimia nervosa rarely occurs before the onset of puberty but may occur in 1–2% of females aged 16–35, and perhaps one thirtieth of this in males.[10,11] The peak age of onset is probably in late adolescence, although binge-eating and vomiting may be kept secret for years, and most cases present in their 20s.

**BOX 28.3** Case Example

At the age of 15 years, Gina is referred by her School Nurse to the Primary Mental Health Worker because she has been found vomiting in the school toilets. Gina has admitted that she occasionally binges and vomits at home.

Gina reveals a bit more to the Primary Mental Health Worker. She has been vomiting after her evening meal without her parents knowing, and binges at times when she is on her own. So she is doing both 10-15 times per week. She is on roughly the 75th centile for both height and weight, with a body mass index of 20.4, just above the 50th centile. Her periods have started to occur irregularly, with a variable amount of bleeding.

*(Continued in Box 28.12)*

In ***binge eating disorder***, the binges are not accompanied by compensatory behaviours or weight and shape concerns, so obesity is likely. This may start in childhood: binge eating has been reported in 6% of children aged six to 13 years (both overweight and normal weight).[12]

***Atypical eating disorder/eating disorder not otherwise specified*** – Epidemiological studies tend to reveal this as the commonest group, but it is really a hotchpotch of different conditions. It includes those that don't fit neatly into the other diagnostic categories – through not meeting all the criteria – because either they have a milder form, are in the early stages, or are partially recovered. This 'condition' can occur as young as six years.[13] With early onset eating disorder traits, it is worth finding out whether the mother has a history of an eating disorder.[14]

**BOX 28.4** Case Example

Henna is 14 years old when her mother takes her to the general practitioner because she is trying to starve herself. She admits to vomiting after meals and occasional binges. She is on the ninth centile for weight and the 50th for height, with a body mass index of 16.2, between the second and ninth centiles. Her periods have become much less frequent during the last six months, and are now occurring once every eight to 10 weeks, the last being three weeks before the appointment.

The general practitioner thinks she has something between anorexia nervosa and bulimia nervosa. He wants to refer her to specialist CAMHS, but Henna refuses, as she does not want to be thought of as mad. The general practitioner bargains with her, and eventually they agree the following:

1 Henna will see the school counsellor, who will report to her parents at least twice a term, mainly to confirm Henna is attending regularly.
2 Henna will be weighed by the practice nurse once every two weeks.
3 If there is a persisting downward trend in her weight, or if her body mass index goes below the second centile (currently 15.6), she will have to accept a referral to specialist CAMHS.

Henna meets with the school counsellor regularly, comes for her regular weighing sessions, and eats enough (and vomits seldom enough) to avoid a referral. At the seventh individual talking session, Henna discloses sexual abuse. She was raped by a 14-year-old boy two years before while camping in Spain with her parents during the summer holidays; they thought she was just spending an evening out with the other teenagers on the campsite. She felt so guilty that she could not tell her parents at the time, but she agrees to allow the counsellor to tell them now. The counsellor also feels obliged to tell social services, which Henna reluctantly accepts, but neither they nor the police can do anything, as Henna does not know the boy's surname or address.

After another term of counselling, Henna is able to tell her general practitioner that she is no longer trying to starve herself or bingeing or vomiting. Her body mass index is 17, on the ninth centile. Her periods have become more regular and frequent. He agrees that she can stop the regular weighing and the counselling if she wants. She meets with the counsellor once a term for the next year, and all remains well.

**BOX 28.5** Case Example

Debbie is eight years old when she tells her parents that she does not want to eat. She does not give any reason except that she is fat. She is slightly overweight. Her parents try for a month to persuade her to eat, but every mealtime is a struggle, and so they take her to the general practitioner.

Assessment by Tier 3 CAMHS is inconclusive. Her weight centile is still a little above her height centile. She is told she will die if she continues to starve herself. She agrees to see the clinic art therapist; her parents see a different CAMHS worker; and there are regular reviews involving all of them.

After a year, Debbie becomes able to eat normally without her parents having to supervise and encourage her closely. The art therapist has reflected to Debbie that some of her artwork makes it look as if she has been sexually abused, but Debbie consistently denies this. With Debbie's permission, her parents have been told of this conjecture, but cannot think of any particular occasion when this might have occurred.

After a further six months, Debbie is discharged, apparently cured of at least her eating disorder.

## Other eating problems
*Food avoidance emotional disorder* – This consists of marked avoidance of food *without* distorted weight and shape cognitions: an affected child knows that she is underweight and would like to be heavier, but may not know why she finds this difficult to achieve.[15] She may be anxious about the consequences of eating: saying for instance that she is afraid of being sick, 'not hungry', 'can't eat' or 'eating hurts my tummy'. It can occur from about the age of six years onwards. Referral to a paediatrician is usually necessary to exclude occasional unidentified organic pathology.

**BOX 28.6** Case Example

Cicely, aged nine years, is referred by her general practitioner to her primary mental health worker because she is afraid to eat. A year ago, she had a viral illness that led to repeated vomiting. She refuses to eat any of the foods that she vomited up then, and is reluctant to eat any new foods, so her intake is limited. She is on the ninth centile for weight and the 50th centile for height, with a body mass index of 13.3, close to the second centile.

The primary mental health worker embarks on a course of anxiety management, with gradual introduction of new foods. After six months, Cicely is eating a much more varied diet, her weight has climbed up to the 25th centile and her body mass index to 14.9, between the ninth and 25th centiles.

One particular anxiety, a fear of choking, can give rise to what used to be called *globus hystericus*, but is now usually called **functional dysphagia**, in which swallowing difficulties are combined with a feeling of tightness in the throat. There may be a history of a particularly traumatic episode of choking or vomiting.

**BOX 28.7** Case Example

Saheeda, aged seven years, choked on a lump of bread during a family meal. Her father did the Heimlich manoeuvre, and she came to no harm, but she subsequently developed a fear of choking again. She is therefore reluctant to eat any lumpy food. A year later, her parents become concerned about her poor growth and ask for help.

**Pervasive refusal syndrome** is a very rare condition occurring in girls of 8–14 years who not only stop eating but also stop drinking, walking, talking or caring for themselves. It seems at least sometimes to be an extreme post-traumatic stress reaction to some form of abuse, and can also be understood as a form of learned helplessness.[16]

The last three conditions are mentioned because they can sometimes cause confusion with anorexia nervosa: they will not be discussed further.

### How do eating disorders develop?

As with many other psychological disorders, both **genetic and environmental factors** contribute to the development of eating disorders.[17] *Rumination* may also play an important role in maintaining the thoughts generating eating-disordered behaviours – meaning a cyclical sequence of thoughts that goes round and round without leading to any new insights (*see* Table 28.1 in Chapter 39 on obsessive-compulsive disorder).

**Genetic factors** – There seems to be shared familial liability between the different eating disorders, implying some genetic influence on the whole group.

There are also some genetic links with obsessional or perfectionist traits and with depression. Relatives of bulimics have a higher rate of substance misuse, especially alcoholism.

*Environmental factors* – Living in a Western society makes an eating disorder more likely to occur: this may be partly due to the worship of thinness that is now part of our culture. For individuals, non-specific factors such as sexual abuse, low self-esteem or anxiety may play an important role. The apparent salience of sexual abuse in those victims who develop eating disorders may be because of its impact on feelings about the self and one's body, and the link between these two. Sexual abuse may lead to avoidance of intimate relationships in some and sexual promiscuity in others; this type of abuse may also contribute to the development of overeating in some and restriction of calories in others – or a combination of the two (or neither).

*Family factors* may (often inadvertently) help to initiate or maintain the young person's eating behaviour, such as:
➤ family dieting
➤ high parental expectations
➤ siblings who are more successful
➤ conflict or inconsistency between parents
➤ parental separation (the eating behaviour can be seen as having the function of keeping the absent parent more involved or bringing the separated parents together)
➤ unsatisfactory contact arrangements
➤ parents who are reluctant to confront the young person's eating behaviour for fear of creating conflict
➤ the eating behaviours becoming a battle of wills with parents that takes on a life of its own (overt if dieting or covert if vomiting or bingeing).

The young person's attitude to food and eating may be significantly affected by critical comments about eating, shape or weight from family members or peers, or by recreational pressure: for instance, girls at ballet school or in competitive sports may be at risk unless they are trained to substantiate their calorie input. More specific factors seem to operate in bulimia, such as family obesity and early menarche, which could have an influence by sensitising the young person to her shape, thereby encouraging dieting. In children and teenagers vulnerable to eating disorders, dieting can become an obsession that takes on a power of its own. This may be more likely in high-achieving or perfectionist individuals. A stint of dieting may be precipitated by an event with an emotional impact, such as: being bullied about being 'fat', being pressurised by peers into becoming thinner, or having a viral infection that transiently diminishes appetite.[18]

*Psychopathology* – In both anorexia and bulimia, there is likely to be intense preoccupation with:
➤ evaluating the self in terms of weight and shape
➤ seeking control of feelings (and even external events) by controlling food intake and weight.

The central importance of *shape* may be reflected in repeated scrutiny of certain parts of the body, such as cheeks, tummy or bottom, which can contribute to over-estimation of *size*. All other personal qualities and attributes are relegated below the belief (which can become religious in quality) that self-worth depends on what weighing scales say, what the mirror reflects, or how successfully food can be avoided in the face of hunger. Going without food is seen as virtuous, as in asceticism, and becomes a form of successful control – and it seems that the achieved 'high' may be more than just the glory of success, as in the religious trances induced by the fasting of the ascetic.

A young person may sometimes describe unwanted emotional states as 'feeling fat' and equate these with actually being fat.[19] Dysfunctional eating can serve a very useful function in processing feelings. Restricting food can regulate uncomfortable feelings such as anxiety or disappointment. Bingeing can fill a void or feeling of emptiness. Vomiting or purging can be a way of expelling or evacuating unwanted feelings. Exercise can induce a strong feeling of well-being and satisfaction. Thus the habits developed as part of an eating disorder may be very rewarding, and may not go away until alternative methods of dealing with emotions can be developed.

To summarise this, the rewards of hunger/starvation/thinness may include:

➤ feeling virtuous
➤ feeling in control
➤ feeling superior to others
➤ feeling attractive to others
➤ feeling full of energy
➤ feeling able to concentrate fully
➤ managing unpleasant emotions.

In anorexia nervosa, there is seldom much motivation to change, since low weight is seen as an accomplishment rather than an affliction: starvation can become more of a pleasure than eating, and may then take on aspects of an addiction. A young person with bulimia nervosa may see herself as a failed anorexic, since her attempts to control shape and weight are undermined by frequent episodes of excessive eating (dyscontrol): her motivation may be to become thinner rather than to stop vomiting.

*Circular causality* may operate here. A young person who develops anorexia is likely to have pre-existing obsessional or perfectionist traits, and is also likely to become more obsessional the more successful her dieting. Success with self-denial and thinness can counteract fragile self-esteem, feelings of ineffectiveness or self-loathing (which may in part explain the occasional association with sexual abuse). At the same time, malnutrition may exacerbate low mood or dysphoria, leading to a vicious circle (*see* Figure 28.1). Interest and involvement with other people declines as the young person loses weight, and she is likely to become socially withdrawn and isolated. Such psychosocial features tend to get worse with weight loss and often improve with weight regain.

A similar pattern of circular causality may characterise **bulimia nervosa**, as shown in Figure 28.2.

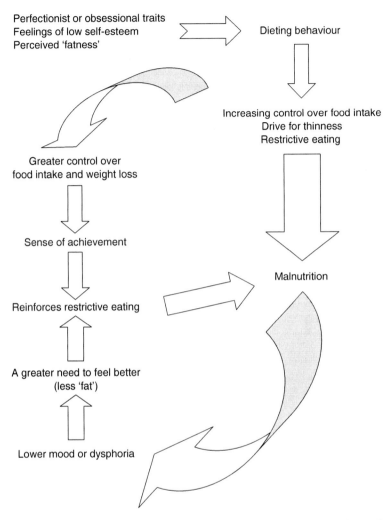

**FIGURE 28.1** An example of circular causality in anorexia nervosa (Note: this is not presented as an all-encompassing model, but merely as one way in which the symptoms of anorexia nervosa can become self-perpetuating.)

These are simplified examples to aid understanding of what can be a complex and varied mix of conscious and unconscious thought patterns, varying from one individual to another. It can be helpful as part of assessment or management to draw an ***individual diagram*** with the young person.

## ASSESSMENT

Early detection is important, as the distorted habits and attitudes to food are easier to shift if recognised soon after they have begun to cause weight loss. If weight loss can be reversed and attitudes shifted *before* the stage when inpatient treatment is required, then the prognosis is likely to be better. Early detection

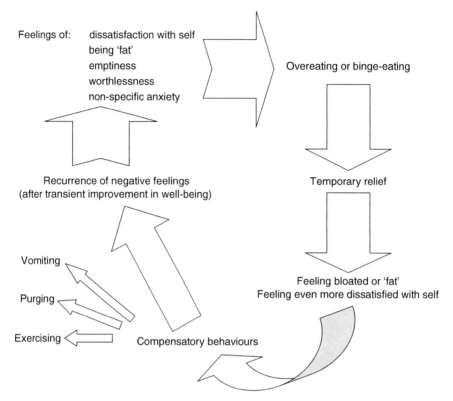

**FIGURE 28.2** An example of circular causality in bulimia nervosa (Note: this is not presented as an all-encompassing model, but merely as one way in which the symptoms of bulimia nervosa can become self-perpetuating.)

in the community is therefore vital, as is a referral pathway for timely specialist assessment.

Indicators of an established eating disorder are:
➤ being underweight
➤ restricting intake
➤ vomiting
➤ bingeing
➤ excessive exercise
➤ an increased need for control
➤ excessive use of laxatives.

Earlier warning signs that a young person may be developing an eating disorder include the following.
➤ Dieting or avoidance of food, often in secret.
➤ Avoidance of eating in front of others.
➤ Preoccupation with food or cooking for others.
➤ Concealing weight loss, for instance by wearing baggy clothes.

➤ Spending an inordinate amount of time after every meal in the bathroom.
➤ Exercising a lot, often in secret.
➤ A reduction in self-esteem or alteration in mood, such as increased depressive feelings.
➤ Overvaluing shape or weight – many adolescent girls are aware that health professionals may ask about distorted body image, so may say initially that they think they are too thin. They may nevertheless be sensitive about body shape or see themselves as too fat, as revealed by comments to friends, or when on a weighing scale or in front of a mirror. Adolescent boys may be more concerned about being muscular, but conflate this with losing fat, rather than realising that not only exercise but also calorie intake need to be increased to sustain big muscles.

Ask a carer whether she is aware of or suspects any of these. Speak to the young person on her own about how she sees herself, her view of the problem, the pressures she is under (for instance at school) and any other worries or concerns she may have. Try to understand what may have led to the development and maintenance of the eating problem. Also ask about obsessional symptoms and mood, as depression and obsessive-compulsive disorder commonly occur in individuals with eating disorders.

Assessment of possible **bulimia nervosa** involves thinking of the possibility, so ask about binge-eating and compensatory behaviours, especially vomiting (which is usually secretive). Frequent vomiting can cause erosion of tooth enamel, low blood potassium and multicystic ovaries, which lead to irregular periods and reduced fertility. It is worth discussing these possibilities, if only to explore motivations to change. It is also worth asking about impulsive risk-taking behaviours.

**BOX 28.8** Alarm Bells in the assessment of an eating disorder

Rapid loss of weight (more than 0.5 kg per week)
Very low intake of energy-dense food
Obsessional or secretive exercising
Frequent visits to the bathroom
Periods becoming irregular or infrequent
Lack of expected gain in height
Weight less than 75% of what it should be for height
Body mass index less than second centile
Intermittent excessive use of alcohol or drugs, including laxatives
Recurrent self-harm (usually cutting)
Persisting low mood

### Differential diagnosis

There are other reasons, both physical and psychological, why a young person may lose weight. Physical causes include hyperthyroidism, diabetes, gastrointestinal problems such as Crohn's disease, or any serious illness. Substance misuse, particularly with amphetamines, can cause significant weight loss. Weight loss can also occur in severe depression, as a result of the low mood. However, starvation can lead to depressive feelings as well as the other way round, so depressive disorder may at times be difficult to differentiate from anorexia nervosa, particularly if the two coexist. The time sequence (which symptoms started first) helps to decide which of these two problems is likely to be primary, as does the relative prominence of the two sets of characteristic symptoms.

### Obesity

As part of the assessment of obesity, it is worth looking at general behavioural issues within the family and in particular how the child is rewarded. Does food play a significant part in reward-giving or enjoyable family activities?

## MANAGEMENT AND REFERRAL[20]

### Selective eating

Monitor the child's weight and linear growth. If this is satisfactory, the growth chart can be used to allay the parents' anxiety. If the child is growing but there are concerns about the adequacy of her nutritional intake, refer to a paediatric dietician. If her growth is falling down through the centiles, or if parental anxiety cannot be assuaged, then refer to a paediatrician, who may in turn refer on to the local specialised CAMHS service.

Relaxation of parental pressure to eat a wider range of foods often results in the child gradually experimenting more widely. Even if he does not, carers can usually come to accept the situation. Established food fads do not respond well to psychological treatments, and it is probably not a good use of resources to attempt to treat selective eating in primary school children. When the child is old enough to want to alter the situation himself, perhaps at 13 or 14, treatment is more likely to work – unless there is an underlying autistic spectrum disorder.

### BOX 28.9 Case Example

Jeremy, aged eight years, will allegedly eat only burgers and chips. When his parents see a paediatric dietician, it becomes clear that he is having cereal for breakfast and is drinking additional milk. He will also eat the occasional apple and tangerine. His growth chart is satisfactory. So despite his limited dietary range, his intake is nutritionally adequate, and his parents agree they will stop punishing Jeremy for not eating vegetables at mealtimes.

### Anorexia nervosa

The importance of early detection means that it is ***everyone's business*** to ensure that recognition and intervention happen as early as possible, including: parents, other carers or family members, teachers, school welfare officers, community school nurses, general practitioners and dieticians. When in doubt, weight and height should be measured and body mass index calculated. Referral should be sooner rather than later, but the initial intervention may be just to monitor weight for a few weeks to establish the trend.

A young person who has not yet seen her *general practitioner* should do so, as she is in the best position to consider the medical seriousness and the possibility of any other medical conditions. Some parents or young people may not immediately accept referral to a mental health service; for these families, initial referral could be to a paediatrician or paediatric dietician.

Once the early stages have been missed, management becomes more challenging. *Acute deterioration* is indicated by:

➤ cold or blue extremities
➤ slow pulse and/or low blood pressure
➤ an increased rate of weight loss
➤ fatigue and lethargy.

This sort of combination needs urgent paediatric referral, with a view to admission to a paediatric ward for further assessment and stabilisation.

A more *chronic presentation* without definite medical complications should be referred direct to specialist CAMHS: most services should have a fast-track referral pathway for suspected anorexia nervosa.

Definite cases of anorexia nervosa, whether acute or chronic, should be managed by specialist CAMHS who may in turn refer on to inpatient services. A recent randomised trial suggested no advantage to inpatient treatment compared to outpatient, and no advantage to specialist Tier 4 outpatient treatment compared to routine Tier 3 CAMHS outpatient treatment.[21] It is therefore logical to keep young people out of hospital and engaged in outpatient treatment packages whenever possible, although the threat of possible admission if weight should plummet may often be a powerful motivator to help engagement with the offered outpatient treatment. Several centres have recently set up trials of multi-family group therapy, a promising innovation that may perhaps reduce the need for inpatient treatment. Inpatient admission should however be arranged if the maximum possible outpatient treatment has not shifted the situation; or if medical complications (such as loss of weight or low potassium) are life-threatening.

The following approaches may be helpful in milder cases or in what seems to be an early stage, or in those more severe cases who have to wait for specialist assessment.

➤ *Increase parental anxiety* – It may *appear* helpful to reassure, but with a potentially life-threatening condition, parents need to be encouraged to worry. Explaining the serious consequences of allowing the weight loss to continue and of not getting appropriate treatment may make it easier for parents to accept a referral to a mental health service.
➤ Parents need to make every effort to be *in charge of the child's eating* (rather than allowing the young person's eating behaviour to be in charge of everyone). If there are two parents or carers, it is essential they work together on

this. It may be more difficult for an unsupported single parent to take charge of the young person's eating behaviour, so single parents should be encouraged to enlist whatever help they can from amongst friends or extended family. The earlier this process starts, the more rapidly it is likely to succeed.

➤ It is not usually necessary to instruct parents in *ways of helping their daughter eat* – they can be remarkably inventive about finding ways of doing this for themselves, given adequate support. They are likely to increase supervision, especially at mealtimes, and may for instance use rewards and sanctions, such as allowing a favourite activity only if a particular meal is eaten. Force-feeding and punitive behavioural methods should be avoided, as they are likely to make the eating disorder worse in the long run.

➤ *Engage the young person* by externalising the problem. Describe the disorder as something that takes people over: it is making her do things she does not really want to do. 'Let's fight the anorexia monster together.'

➤ *Dietary management.* Referral to a paediatric dietician can be very useful to assess current calorie intake, and for advice on a sensible eating regime. Dietary supplements such as Fortisip may be helpful as an additional source of calories, but if they are instead used as an alternative to eating food, then they will not increase overall calorie intake, and so may give a false sense that something has been achieved.

**BOX 28.10** Case Example

Jemima, aged 14-and-a-half years, is brought to her general practitioner by her mother, with a four-month history of loss of weight and decreasing food intake. Her height is on the 75th centile and her weight on the 25th centile, giving her a weight for height of 85% and a body mass index of 17.1, just above the ninth centile.

She says that she has been teased by someone at school about her weight, and several friends are on diets: she is the most successful. She reluctantly admits that, despite recent weight loss, she still thinks she is too fat. She also admits to doing press-ups in her room every evening, but not to bingeing, vomiting or using laxatives. Her periods started 18 months ago, and were initially regular, but the last one was three months ago. She has no boyfriend. (Community school nursing records subsequently show that her weight was on the 90th centile at secondary school entry.)

The general practitioner explains to the girl that she has been overtaken by ideas about dieting that are making her go too far – overshoot the mark – so that she cannot stop getting thinner. She is in danger of becoming dangerously thin, and, if she continues to lose weight, would probably have to go to hospital, and certainly have to see a child psychiatrist. Jemima's mother is not happy about this, but is appropriately concerned, and agrees to bring her husband to an evening appointment two weeks later. The general practitioner also sends Jemima to the local dietician, who judges her oral intake to be 900 calories per day, and advises it should instead be 2 000 calories per day, giving suggestions to her mother on how to achieve this.

With the parents on their own, the general practitioner explains his concern that their daughter is developing anorexia nervosa. He goes on to describe the implications of continued weight loss, and the life-threatening nature of the disorder if it is allowed to become severe. He invites them to think of ways in which they could be firm about encouraging her to eat. The parents brainstorm this problem and generate some solutions. For instance, Jemima loves horse-riding and would like to go to the stables every evening: her parents decide they will let her go only if they have observed her eating what the dietician has described as an adequate meal.

Fortnightly weights show an initial weight gain, which then slows. Appointments with the dietician are reduced from fortnightly to monthly, and reviews by the general practitioner are reduced from monthly to every two months. Six months later, the girl's periods restart, but she still thinks she is too fat for at least part of the time, in spite of being on the 50th centile for weight and 90% of ideal weight for height, with a body mass index of 19.2, between the 25th and 50th centiles.

## Bulimia nervosa

A teenager often does not present for help with symptoms of bingeing and vomiting until she is no longer a teenager. She may be unwilling to let her parents or anyone else know the full extent of her symptoms, and may be ambivalent about seeking help. This can make any form of treatment problematic, particularly family therapy. *Individual therapy* has been shown successful in clinical trials in adults – specifically cognitive-behavioural therapy and interpersonal therapy – but it is not always easy to engage a young person in a prolonged period of self-reflection if she sees little reason to change.[22] The therapeutic discussion may for instance focus on food, and the thoughts and feelings linked to food, as in cognitive-behavioural therapy, or focus on relationships and their links to feelings, without any discussion of food, as in interpersonal therapy. Adolescent counselling services, for instance provided by charitable organisations, may be able to provide this.

Advice about medical complications can also be useful as a form of *psychoeducation*, although it is uncertain how often it may increase motivation to change. Vomiting or laxative use can be life-threatening if it is frequent enough for the serum potassium to drop below normal. Teenagers are often impressed by stories of rotting tooth enamel, and a visit to the dentist should be encouraged. There may be cystic changes in the ovaries leading to reduced egg quality and therefore reduced fertility. If any of these seems likely, for instance if vomiting is occurring more than three times per day, it is worth arranging for a medical opinion from a general practitioner or paediatrician, with a view to appropriate blood tests and if possible an ovarian ultrasound.

For a teenager who genuinely wants help, referral should be made to a relevant *counselling* service or specialist CAMHS for appropriate individual therapy and possibly other interventions, such as group work or family work. Providing assessment has been done and counselling is available, *medication* may be considered.

Fluoxetine (20–60 mg per day, in a single morning dose) may provide a short-term reduction in bingeing and vomiting,[23] but will probably have no impact on the underlying cognitions.

**BOX 28.11** Summary points about anorexia nervosa

Anorexia nervosa can begin as young as eight.

Anorexia nervosa can occur in boys as well as girls.

Attitudes to food and fatness are more extreme than in other causes of weight loss.

It may present with failure to follow centiles, rather than actual weight loss.

The parents need to be in control of their child's tendency to eat too little. The earlier this happens in the course of the disease, the better the prognosis.

Successful management can be relatively straightforward if the condition is recognised early enough.

Whether referring or not, plot a growth chart and calculate body mass index.

**BOX 28.12** Case Example continued from Box 28.3

The primary mental health worker asks 15-year-old Gina what she wants to do about her bingeing and vomiting. Gina says she can manage things all on her own, doesn't want her parents to know, and certainly does *not* want any 'counselling'. The primary mental health worker asks Gina if she understands what makes the frequency of bingeing and particularly vomiting so worrying for professionals. It is clear that Gina does not, so the primary mental health worker explains the medical consequences detailed in the related paragraph on psychoeducation.

Gina agrees to ask her dentist, whom she happens to be seeing for a check-up within the next few weeks, about her tooth enamel. She reluctantly agrees to her parents being told – in her presence. But she refuses any tests or referral to a general practitioner, paediatrician or psychiatrist and says she does not want to talk to anyone about her issues.

The primary mental health worker succeeds in arranging a meeting with both Gina's parents. By agreement, she has not told Gina's parents what the meeting is about, but has left this to Gina. She meets with Gina before meeting with her parents to negotiate again what she can tell them. Gina says she has already told them all the essential details, but on further questioning admits that she has mentioned the bingeing, which her parents had already suspected from the increased supermarket bills, but has not discussed the vomiting. The primary mental health worker insists that Gina's parents must be told about this, because of its dangers, and Gina acquiesces.

When the four of them meet together, Gina's parents are shocked and concerned to hear of Gina's vomiting and its frequency, but react calmly without becoming angry with her for keeping this a secret. To everyone's surprise, Gina bursts into tears at their reaction, and says she wishes she did not have to fill up her emptiness with food she does not really want.

After a prolonged discussion, some agreements are reached. It emerges that Gina would like to be able to talk more to her parents, although she does not think her friends would see this as 'cool'. Gina's mother says she will set aside a time each weekday evening for Gina to talk to her about whatever she wants. Gina's father says he will give up one of his weekend golfing sessions to go on countryside walks with Gina, which she agrees she would like: he points out that there is no need to talk about anything if she would prefer to remain silent.

At the agreed three-month follow-up appointment, Gina admits she is still binge-ing and vomiting, but now less than once a day. Her dentist, on prompting, has noted that she already has some erosion of her tooth enamel. She has been able to spend more time with her parents, and sometimes can confide in them some of the things that get to her, in relation for instance to her schoolwork, her friends and her younger sister. She also now has a supportive boyfriend to whom she finds it very easy to talk; on her mother's advice, she has not allowed him to induce her to give up all her female friends. It is clear that with all this support, she has no need of counselling. What is less clear is how her bulimic symptoms may develop over time.

Gina agrees with the primary mental health worker and her parents that they will not make any further appointments at present, but that she may need to seek help in the future, for instance if her bulimic symptoms were to become a problem at university.

**BOX 28.13** Summary points about bulimia nervosa and binge eating

Bulimia nervosa rarely begins before puberty, although binge eating often does.
Secrecy is characteristic – especially about vomiting.
A normal weight or underweight bulimic is likely to be a successful vomiter.
In contrast, a binge eater is usually overweight.
A subgroup of bulimics have multi-impulsive behaviours such as cutting, substance misuse, binge-drinking or promiscuous sexual behaviour.
Engagement with professionals is usually necessary for any improvement in symp-toms to occur.
Explaining about medical complications may help (or may not).

## Obesity

Obese children are usually fat because their intake of calories is more than their expenditure. While genetic factors may be relevant, and family eating habits invar-iably are, endocrine causes are rare. One of the conditions predisposing to the most severe obesity is Prader-Willi syndrome, which should be diagnosed in the early years of life through chromosome analysis, because of dysmorphic features and floppiness. Other syndromes are probably even rarer. Low self-esteem and other psychological problems are common, but it is not easy to tell whether they are the cause or the consequence of the obesity.

**Psychoeducation** is of dubious value. Warning adolescents of future health risks is probably counterproductive. A pre-adolescent child is unlikely to care about consequences she sees as so far in the future. Parents have the right to be informed of potential health risks, such as early death, diabetes and high blood pressure, but this by itself is unlikely to change parental or child behaviour.

Recommended treatment for childhood obesity includes the following components.

➤ A balanced, healthy diet – calorie reductions can be achieved by eliminating takeaway and ready prepared foods, which tend to be particularly energy dense, and by limiting portion sizes. Limiting eating to mealtimes, and avoiding high fat snacks such as crisps and biscuits and high-sugar drinks, may also help

➤ An equal emphasis on exercise

➤ A goal of gradual weight loss, of about 0.5 kg per week

➤ Parental support

➤ Behaviour therapy for both child and parents to achieve the diet and exercise goals

➤ Enrolment in a supportive club that involves some form of group exercise

➤ General behavioural advice

➤ Changing any behavioural rewards that include food to ones that don't.

In some cases, this programme may be best organised by a paediatric dietician and/or an interested paediatrician. In the long term, primary care professionals have a major role to play in helping to shape a family's attitudes to food from the birth of the first child onwards.

## RESOURCES
### Websites
- The UK Eating Disorders Association is called 'b-eat' or just 'beat'. Their Helpline is available at 0845 634 1414, and their Youthline is 0845 634 7650. www.b-eat.co.uk/Home
- MEND (Mind, Exercise, Nutrition . . . Do it!) is a social enterprise dedicated to reducing global overweight and obesity levels by helping children and their families become fitter, healthier and happier through offering free healthy living programmes in the local community. www.mendprogramme.org/home

### Growth charts
- BMI growth charts are produced by the Child Growth Foundation and can be obtained from Harlow Healthcare on: http://shop.healthforallchildren.co.uk/pro.epl?DO=PRODUCT& WAY=INFO&ID=224

### Books for young people
- Chilman-Blair K, Taddeo J. *What's Up with Paris? Medikidz explain childhood overweight.* London: Medikidz Publishing; 2009.
  This graphic novel explains the medical aspects of obesity by taking Paris to a tour of Medi-land, a distant planet whose geography and inhabitants bear a striking similarity to the

intricacies of human anatomy and physiology. Along the way she dodges teeth the size of buildings, braves the corrosive waters of the stomach and – yes – learns to control her weight.
- Cooper P. *Overcoming Bulimia Nervosa and Binge-Eating.* London: Robinson; 2009.
- Freeman C. *Overcoming Anorexia Nervosa.* London: Robinson; 2009.
- Schmidt U, Treasure J. *Getting Better Bit(e) by Bit(e): survival kit for sufferers of bulimia nervosa and binge eating disorders.* London: Psychology Press; 1993.
  A self-help book which empowers sufferers (young and old) to take control of their own lives and tackle their eating difficulties.
- Wilson J. *Girls Under Pressure.* London: Corgi Children's; 2007. Feeling as if she doesn't measure up to her 'drop-dead gorgeous' friends, Ellie tries to take control of her weight, and end ups battling with bulimia.

## Reading for parents
- Royal College of Psychiatrists: Mental Health and Growing Up. 3rd ed. Factsheet 24: for parents and teachers: eating disorders in young people; Factsheet 35: for young people: worries about weight. www.rcpsych.ac.uk/mentalhealthinformation/mentalhealthandgrowingup.aspx
- Treasure J, Smith G, Crane A. *Skills-based Learning for Caring for a Loved One with an Eating Disorder: the new Maudsley method.* London: Routledge; 2007.
- Two small booklets giving convenient basic information called: *All about anorexia nervosa* and *All about Bulimia Nervosa* from the Mental Health Foundation are available to download free from:
  www.mhf.org.uk/publications/?EntryId=43109
  www.mhf.org.uk/publications/?EntryId=43112
- Fox C, Joughin C. *Eating Problems in Children: information for parents.* London: Gaskell (Royal College of Psychiatrists); 2002.
- This guide tackles issues such as the different types of eating disorders children can suffer from, how common they are, what causes them, the types of treatment available and the long-term outlook.
- Abraham S. *Eating Disorders (The Facts).* Oxford: Oxford University Press; 2008. This is a comprehensive guide to anorexia nervosa, bulimia nervosa and obesity.

## REFERENCES

1 Stein A, Woolley H, McPherson K. Conflict between mothers with eating disorders and their infants during mealtimes. *Br J Psychiatry.* 1999; **175**(11): 455–61.
2 Fairburn CG, Harrison PJ. Eating disorders. *Lancet.* 2003; **361**(9355): 407–16.
3 Nicholls D, Bryant-Waugh R. Eating disorders of infancy and childhood: definition, symptomatology, epidemiology, and comorbidity. *Child Adolesc Psychiatr Clin N Am.* 2009; **18**(1): 17–30.
4 Lask B, Bryant-Waugh R, editors. *Eating Disorders in Childhood and Adolescence.* 3rd ed. Hove: Psychology Press; 2007.
5 Nicholls DE, Lynn R, Viner RM. Childhood eating disorders: British national surveillance study. *Br J Psychiatry.* 2011; **198**(4): 295–301.
6 Nicholls, 2009, op. cit.
7 Nicholls, 2007, op. cit.
8 Fairburn, op. cit.
9 Gowers SG. Management of eating disorders in children and adolescents. *Arch Dis Child.* 2008; **93**: 331–4.

10 Nicholls. 2007, op. cit.

11 Fairburn, op. cit.

12 Nicholls, 2009, op. cit.

13 Nicholls, 2007, op. cit.

14 Stein A, Woolley H, Cooper S, *et al.* Eating habits and attitudes among 10-year-old children of mothers with eating disorders: longitudinal study. *Br J Psychiatry.* 2006; **189**(10): 324–9.

15 Nicholls, 2009, op. cit.

16 Nicholls, 2009, op. cit.

17 Fairburn, op. cit.

18 Park RJ. Lawrie SM, Freeman CP. Post-viral onset of anorexia nervosa. *Br J Psychiatry.* 1995; **166**(3): 386–9.

19 Gowers, op. cit.

20 National Collaborating Centre for Mental Health. *Eating Disorders: core interventions in the treatment and management of anorexia nervosa, bulimia nervosa and related eating disorders* [NICE clinical guideline number 9]. London: National Institute for Health and Clinical Excellence; 2004.

21 Gowers SG, Clark A, Roberts C, *et al.* Clinical effectiveness of treatments for anorexia nervosa in adolescents: randomised controlled trial. *Br J Psychiatry.* 2007; **91**: 427–35.

22 Gowers, op. cit.

23 NICE, 2004, op. cit.

# CHAPTER 29

# Chronic fatigue syndrome/myalgic encephalomyelitis[1]

## INTRODUCTION

Is this condition a mental health problem at all? Probably not. Unfortunately for sufferers, an exact cause has yet to be identified: once it has, it will be much easier to think of affected young people as suffering from a chronic illness with associated psychosocial morbidity. At present, some of this morbidity arises from professionals appearing to the family to disbelieve that the condition is real. There is a potentially confusing relationship between symptoms of fatigue and symptoms of anxiety or depression,[2] one component of which seems to be that the psychological and physical symptoms each make the other worse. Some professionals erroneously deduce from the evident efficacy of treatments with a strong psychological component (such as graded exercise treatment and cognitive behavioural therapy) that not only maintaining factors but also causative factors *must* include a significant psychological component.[3]

**BOX 29.1** Case Example

A seven-year-old boy is referred for help to a child psychiatrist regarding the boy's increasing symptoms of fatigue. The psychiatrist's comments imply to his mother an element of disbelief. He explores the family history and then recommends some work on the mother-child relationship. The mother refuses to return there, but insists on a referral to a paediatrician, who does a thorough assessment and makes a diagnosis of myalgic encephalomyelitis. Although it takes two years for the fatigue to subside, the boy and his mother are much happier with this approach.

## ASSESSMENT

### Definitions

The terminology for this condition is almost as controversial as its nature and management. Although many professionals prefer the term 'chronic fatigue syndrome' (CFS), and this is the term used most consistently in the medical literature, many sufferers and patients' organisations prefer the term 'ME', which can mean either myalgic encephalomyelitis or myalgic encephalopathy. Professionals prefer a term that does not make implications about aetiology; whereas sufferers and their families prefer a term that implies an organic cause, albeit unknown, and shy away from a term that seems uncomfortably vague and could be taken to imply that the illness is primarily psychological. We have decided to follow the Royal College of Paediatrics and Child Health[4] and NICE[5] in hedging our bets, so we use the combined acronym CFS/ME.

Four possible definitions are shown in Table 29.1 (with some wording slightly altered).[6,7,8] We do not want to get bogged down by a discussion about terminology, but any diagnosis that relies too much on excluding other conditions is inherently unsatisfactory, since updates in medical knowledge may reveal conditions that were not previously (easily) diagnosable, and the emphasis on not being able to find a cause implies misleadingly that there *is* no cause. The definitions were mainly designed for adults, so need to be adapted slightly for children. In particular, the requirement for six months' duration is usually waived in children,[9] and even three months may be too long to wait before allowing a diagnosis. One of the key features in children is fatigability, meaning that the sensation of being tired is exacerbated by any physical or mental exertion, as well as by any infectious illness such as a common cold. In fact physical or mental exertion can make *any* of the symptoms worse, and the child's daily life is intermittently or continuously disrupted, particularly in relation to school attendance or activity.

The diagnosis should ideally be made by a paediatrician, but general practitioners can have an important role in thinking of the diagnosis and making early referrals. The diagnosis should be considered in any child or young person who has had generalised fatigue causing significant impairment for more than three months, and for which no alternative explanation has been found. It appears that the condition can affect children of all ages, at least down to the age of two years, with a frequency that increases with age, but no substantial difference in symptom patterns.[10] The associated symptoms listed in Table 29.1 enable a pattern to be perceived that can establish a positive diagnosis, rather than a diagnosis of exclusion. In some cases, the history suggests that the symptoms have started after a viral infection, but it is not always possible to confirm this by laboratory tests. Evidence for infectious agents as a frequent cause is controversial.[11]

### Epidemiology, aetiology, course and prognosis
Prevalence rates vary because of changing definitions, but for adolescents they are probably in the 50–100 per 100 000 range.[12] Girls appear to be more often affected than boys. It is probably best at present to regard the cause as unknown, but engagement with families is likely to be easier if some physiological or biological origin is assumed.

There is a wide range in the severity of presentation. This ranges from a child who is tired for a few months and has given up sport to a young person who has been bed-bound in a darkened room for three years and may require tube-feeding. Similarly, there is a wide range in the outcome; although the natural course of the

**TABLE 29.1** Definitions of chronic fatigue syndrome or myalgic encephalomyelitis

### National Institute for Health and Clinical Excellence (2007)

*Fatigue* must have all of the following features:
- new or with a specific onset (in other words, it is not lifelong)
- persistent and/or recurrent
- unexplained by other conditions
- resulting in a substantial reduction in activity level, which is characterised by post-exertional malaise and/or fatigue which has:
  - a delayed onset (for example by at least 24 hours)
  - a slow recovery over several days.

*Plus* one or more of the following symptoms:
- difficulty with sleeping, such as:
  - insomnia
  - hypersomnia
  - unrefreshing sleep
  - a disturbed sleep-wake cycle.
- multi-site muscle and/or joint pain not accompanied by signs of inflammation
- headaches
- painful lymph nodes without pathological enlargement
- sore throat
- cognitive dysfunction, such as:
  - difficulty thinking, organising thoughts, planning or processing information
  - inability to concentrate
  - impairment of short-term memory
  - difficulties with word-finding.
- general malaise or 'flu-like' symptoms
- dizziness
- nausea
- palpitations in the absence of identified cardiac pathology
- symptoms worsened by physical or mental exertion.

A minimum of *three months'* fatigue is required before a diagnosis is made.

### Royal College of Paediatrics and Child Health (2004)

*Generalised fatigue* persisting after routine tests and investigations have failed to identify an obvious underlying cause

### Centers for Disease Control and Prevention (1994)

*Four* symptoms are required from the following list:
- substantial impairment in short-term memory or concentration
- sore throat
- tender lymph nodes
- muscle pain
- multi-joint pain without swelling or redness
- headaches of a new type, pattern or severity
- unrefreshing sleep
- post-exertional malaise lasting for longer than 24 hours.

*Fatigue* must have been present for a minimum of six months, and must be:
- clinically evaluated
- unexplained
- persistent or relapsing
- new or have a definite onset (not lifelong)
- not the result of ongoing exertion
- not substantially relieved by rests
- resulting in substantial reduction in previous levels of occupational, educational, social or personal activities.

Conditions that *exclude* the diagnosis include:
- clinically important impairment of physical health
- clinically important impairment of mental health, including major depression, bipolar disorder, psychosis or an eating disorder
- substance misuse.

**Oxford criteria (1991)**

Fatigue must be:
- the principal symptom
- with a definite onset and not lifelong
- severe and disabling fatigue affecting physical and mental functioning.

The fatigue should have been present for a minimum of six months, during which it was present for more than 50% of the time.
Other symptoms could be associated with the main symptom of fatigue, such as myalgia, joint pains, headache and sleep disturbance.
Conditions that *exclude* the diagnosis:
A. Patients with established medical conditions known to produce chronic fatigue.
B. Patients with a current diagnosis of schizophrenia, substance abuse, manic depressive illness, eating disorders and organic brain syndrome. (Note that depression and anxiety are *not* excluded, as they often co-exist with CFS/ME.)

disease is usually to improve with time, and most children recover at least partially, there are a few children who do not seem to get better, and for whom there seems to be no effective treatment. It is therefore foolhardy to predict the course in an individual case, but it does seem likely that children who present at an early stage with a willingness to try offered treatments may get better more quickly.

## The mental health component

The majority of parents with a child afflicted by this puzzling condition prefer to remain under the care of the paediatrician who has made the diagnosis, and resent care being transferred to a psychologist or psychiatrist. For instance, many parents fear that professionals (including paediatricians) do not 'believe in' ME, think it does not have an organic cause, think it is 'all in the mind', or even think that some of the symptoms are made up! A referral to a psychiatrist or psychologist may confirm such suspicions. The 'psycho-person' may explore attitudes and beliefs, and suggest therapy based on thoughts and behaviours, when all the young person and parents want is to target the physical symptoms and get them better. Parents may, however, tolerate a mental health professional as part of the paediatric team.

Nevertheless, it often seems in the authors' view that the physiotherapist or occupational therapist may be in the best position to carry out any psychological therapy. This is because a gradual increase in level of exercise is one of the most effective components of treatment and these professionals are often more easily accepted by the child and her family.

Assessment of psychological well-being is important for young people with CFS/ME, for two reasons: differential diagnosis and comorbidity. Conditions that may cause similar symptoms include anxiety, depressive disorder and school refusal – all three of which commonly occur in children with CFS/ME (without excluding the CFS/ME diagnosis). Other mental health consequences include somatisation and social withdrawal. Personality features that may pre-date the condition, or become more prominent as a consequence, include conscientiousness, vulnerability, a sense of worthlessness and emotional lability.[13]

Attitudinal factors may be an important part of the disease process, whether as consequences or as contributors to its development. Young people with CFS/ME and their parents may have higher expectations of activity levels and be less tolerant of fatigue symptoms compared to controls.[14] Parents of children and young people with CFS/ME may have less belief in psychological contributing factors than matched controls and more belief in constitutional or environmental factors. Children and young people with CFS/ME may be more likely to use an emotional language that emphasises physical symptoms than an emotional language that emphasises internal states or feelings.[15,16,17] The attitude of healthcare professionals may also contribute to the disease: dismissive and unhelpful responses may contribute to a sense of isolation, demoralisation and hopelessness.[18]

## Management

If a mental health professional is to be involved at all (and many parents would prefer not) then this is probably best as part of a team, probably led by a paediatrician. As with many other conditions described in this book, the way in which services are delivered may vary greatly.

The **two main strands** of the management of CFS/ME target activity and sleep. The two are related because fatigue during the day inhibits activity, which leads to difficulty getting to sleep at night, which results in sleep-onset time becoming later and later (delayed sleep phase), which leads to delayed waking the next morning, and so a vicious cycle develops. Sleep quality is often poor, with frequent waking and difficulty getting back to sleep, as is seen commonly in adolescent depression (this sort of sleep disturbance is one of the overlapping symptoms between the two conditions, and can at times cause diagnostic confusion). Daytime fatigue is exacerbated by inadequate sleep, and the young person often stays up into the early hours of the next morning to extract some value from the day. Thus daytime activity cannot be increased without tackling sleep, but sleep onset and quality may remain a problem while activity levels are very low. *See* Figure 29.1.

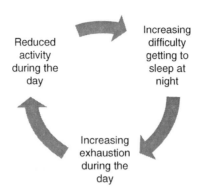

**FIGURE 29.1** The cycle relating activity and sleep

### Addressing sleep and activity

*Sleep hygiene* must be in place: this means common-sense measures to make it easier to go to sleep (*see* Table 36.4: Sleep management tips). The natural tendency for many teenagers, without some over-riding imperative (such as school) to get them out of bed in the morning, is to sleep progressively later in the morning and stay awake progressively later at night. This is particularly likely to occur in CFS/ME. There may be a useful analogy here to experiments involving people who volunteer to stay in an underground cave for extended periods: without cues about daylight rhythms, the natural tendency is for the daily cycle to last 25 hours rather than 24. This may be partly why it seems to be more difficult to make the time of sleep onset and morning waking progressively earlier (which would be analogous to imposing a 23-hour day). It is generally easier to make everything progressively later, and then stop when a socially acceptable timetable has been achieved. So, for instance, a young person who has got into the rhythm of going to sleep at 05.00 and waking at 13.00 is likely to find it easier to shift these times forwards by an hour or half an hour every day than to shift them backwards.

Behavioural measures should be tried first, such as these gradual timetable shifts and the other sleep hygiene measures in Table 36.4; but *medication* may be required, particularly if sleep disturbance is as extreme and intractable as it sometimes can be in CFS/ME.[19] In most cases, melatonin would be the first line; as a more powerful option, low dose tricyclic antidepressants can be very helpful, such as amitriptyline at a dose between 10 and 50 mg. There must be thorough discussion of the risk of overdose. Antihistamines such as promethazine 25 mg may be a useful alternative, although in some children these can cause agitation or nightmares.

*A baseline activity diary* is a useful starting point for a gradual increase in activity. Functionality can be graded each day, using for instance a 0–10 scale, with 10 as 'The most fatigued you could imagine being' and zero as 'The most energetic you could imagine being'. *Activities* can be *physical*, e.g. walking; *mental*, e.g. reading, doing schoolwork; and *social*, e.g. telephoning or meeting friends. *See* Table 29.2.

Once a baseline is established, a programme of regular rest and activities can be agreed. Graded exercise programmes, which may be more acceptable if called '*pacing*', have been shown to be effective in adults, whereas prolonged rest has been

**TABLE 29.2** Example of an activity diary

| Week beginning ...../...../..... | Sunday | Monday | Tuesday | Wednesday | Thursday | Friday | Saturday |
|---|---|---|---|---|---|---|---|
| Fatigue score* | | | | | | | |
| Physical activities | | | | | | | |
| Mental activities | | | | | | | |
| Social activities | | | | | | | |
| Percent of activity target achieved[#] | | | | | | | |

\* Use a 0–10 scale: 10 is the most fatigued you could imagine being and 0 is the most energetic you could imagine being.

[#] Once targets are set, leave blank for a baseline diary.

found to worsen fatigue.[20] Some of the activities revealed on the baseline diary can be gradually increased, whilst ensuring that goals are agreed by the young person and caregivers, and are small and achievable. The young person should be instructed *not* to push herself too hard, and there should be no connotation of forcing her through some sort of pain barrier. Activity targets can be set for each day, and their success rated on the diary. The plotting of improvement in the activity diary will give the responsibility and control to the child or young person, and a sense of achievement, assisting motivation. Young people should be told not to overdo the activity on days when they feel better, but also to try to maintain their levels of activity on days when they feel worse. The pattern to aim for is a gradual trend in increasing overall activity levels. It is important not to set the goals too high, and also to anticipate that there will be ups and downs.

One of the characteristics of CFS/ME is irregular but fairly frequent **relapses** and remissions, perhaps due to an intercurrent infection, or for unknown reasons. The relapses should not be taken to imply that treatment is not working. To avoid despondency, blame and demands for a change of treatment plan, it is important to *predict* that relapses will occur, and *agree* with the young person and caregivers a *strategy for dealing with them*. This should include allowing the young person, with the agreement of carers, to make adjustments in the activity targets: lower targets should be set if it is clear a relapse is beginning, to ensure these are achievable. It is important if possible to keep the activity diary going, with daily ratings of functionality. Table 29.3 shows a hypothetical example of ratings made over a month. Note that fatigue scores are high at the start of the month, so the activity goals are reduced, and ratings of the percentage achieved go up. After two weeks, the fatigue scores have come down, so the activity goals are increased, and the achievement percentages go down a little. After another 10 days, the fatigue scores are higher again, and the activity goals are adjusted downwards, enabling higher percentages of success to be attained. A similar pattern continues for a second month, and the two months are plotted on Figure 29.2, with the scales equalised by multiplying the fatigue score by 10.

An up-and-down pattern is to be expected. Young people and their families need to be supported through each downturn and enabled to extract a small amount of progress from each upturn – but setting expectations too high is probably unhelpful. In this example, it can be seen that the general trend of fatigue scores is downward, though the plot might need to be continued for several months to confirm this. The activity scores do not show such a clear trend, as they are repeatedly adjusted to allow for the current status of fatigue. Management should be directed at an overall gradual decrease in fatigue and increase in activity levels, and adjusted if the trend appears to be less positive than in the example shown. A downward trend may result from the young person trying to do too much too fast.

**BOX 29.2** Issues to address in the management of CFS/ME

Resetting sleep routine
Small-step increases in activity
Predicting and managing relapse
Diet
Pain
Low mood
School attendance
Information
Complementary therapy

**TABLE 29.3** A month's figures from an activity diary

| Day | 1 | 2 | 3 | 4 | 5 | 6 | 7 | 8 | 9 | 10 | 11 | 12 | 13 | 14 | 15 | 16 | 17 | 18 | 19 | 20 | 21 | 22 | 23 | 24 | 25 | 26 | 27 | 28 | 29 | 30 |
|---|---|---|---|---|---|---|---|---|---|---|---|---|---|---|---|---|---|---|---|---|---|---|---|---|---|---|---|---|---|---|
| Fatigue score | 10 | 9 | 8 | 9 | 7 | 7 | 6 | 7 | 6 | 5 | 5 | 4 | 5 | 4 | 5 | 4 | 6 | 5 | 6 | 7 | 7 | 8 | 9 | 9 | 9 | 9 | 8 | 7 | 7 | 6 |
| Percent of activity target achieved | 20 | 50 | 67 | 50 | 80 | 85 | 90 | 85 | 90 | 95 | 95 | 100 | 95 | 100 | 70 | 75 | 67 | 70 | 60 | 50 | 40 | 30 | 20 | 10 | 50 | 50 | 67 | 75 | 75 | 80 |

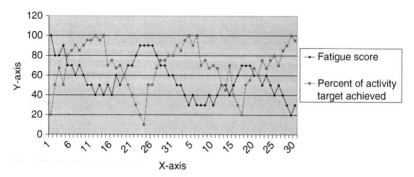

**FIGURE 29.2** Plot of a hypothetical sequence of fatigue and activity scores. X-axis-Date of the month; Y-axis-The fatigue scores have been multiplied by 10 to put them on the same scale as the achievement scores

### Addressing issues other than sleep and activity

General principles suggest that a **balanced diet** will help recovery. The aim should be a regular intake of calories commensurate with the level of activity, including at least the regular daily allowances of vitamins and minerals. Nausea and loss of appetite may make this hard to achieve. The services of a paediatric dietician may be invaluable for detailed advice.

*Pain management* can be a challenge, as some young people with CFS/ME suffer from severe joint and muscle pain of unclear origin. Simple analgesics such as paracetamol or ibuprofen may be sufficient. Second-line measures may include: relaxation and meditation; amitriptyline at a dose of 10–50 mg at night; nortriptyline 10–50 mg at night; involvement of a psychologist to develop strategies for dealing with the pain; or referral to a pain clinic.

If *low mood* is thought to be significantly impairing recovery, whether or not there is a diagnosable major depressive disorder (*see* Chapter 26), then some form of talking therapy should be suggested. This may not be acceptable to the young person or parents, so a full explanation of why this may be beneficial should be given. Antidepressants should be discussed, since they may assist progress. The first-line treatment should be fluoxetine 20 mg, as tricyclics in antidepressant doses (100–150 mg of amitriptyline or nortriptyline) increase the risk of overdose, which is more likely as depression starts to improve. Tricyclics can be very dangerous in overdose, but fluoxetine is entirely safe. Fluoxetine should be started at half the adult dose (10 mg in 2.5 mL of liquid – children below 13 years may need to start on a smaller dose); after about three weeks, if side effects are tolerated, the dose should be increased (unless it is already effective) to the full adult dose (20 mg). It should be reviewed after an initial six-week period on the full dose, when the dose could be further increased (up to a maximum of 60 mg). If successful, the effective dose should be continued for a minimum of six months. It can also help any symptoms of **anxiety** that are present. If side effects or a lack of efficacy dictate a change of medication, then sertraline or citalopram are alternatives.

Anxiety, more often covert than overt, is particularly likely in relation to social contact or **school attendance**. As with other forms of activity, increases in social interaction should be carefully planned and adjusted slowly. If school attendance is an issue, which it is in the majority of cases of CFS/ME, it is essential to obtain the cooperation of school staff in allowing *part-time attendance* and a *reduced level of academic expectation*. School attendance may need to be mornings only, or even single lessons only, initially. Tuition at home or in an undemanding tutorial centre may be necessary.

*Information* about the condition, particularly obtained from the Internet, may occasionally be confusing, so should if possible be discussed. There may be suggestions that professionals mostly do not understand ME, which may be to some extent true, and can be a difficult belief to counter. One way of dealing with it is to acknowledge that most professionals find CFS/ME baffling, but show that nevertheless you know of management strategies that can be effective.

CFS/ME can be an extremely isolating illness, especially for young people who cannot attend school or manage social activities, so **patient support groups** may provide valuable contact with similar aged patients and their parents.

Parents who wish to try **complementary therapies**, such as homoeopathy, can possibly be encouraged, providing they do not spend all the family's savings on expensive unproven treatments, or engage in potentially harmful practices such as colonic washouts or extreme dietary exclusion.[21] Trying too many different interventions at the same time could make it impossible to tell whether any of them are helping.

## REFERRAL

Specialist multidisciplinary teams have been built up in various parts of England since 2004, so referral to these or their satellite teams may be an option for some general practitioners or general paediatricians. Ideally, all but the very mildest cases of CFS/ME should be under the care of a paediatrician (generalist or specialist). If there is no local multidisciplinary team, referral to a local occupational therapist or physiotherapist may be a good way of encouraging a graded increase in activity levels. If the family has fallen out with their paediatrician, the general practitioner will need to be involved in obtaining a second opinion. Shared care (between hospital and primary care) may be necessary at the severe end of the spectrum.

**BOX 29.3** Case Example

Thirteen-year-old Jeremy's parents bring him to their general practitioner for the second time in two months. They inform the general practitioner in no uncertain terms that they will not go back to see the child psychologist. For four months, Jeremy has been suffering from such bad fatigue that he cannot get out of bed until midday and is missing a high proportion of school days. Two months ago, the general practitioner referred him to a consultant paediatrician, who saw him twice and then referred him to a clinical psychologist. The family have fallen out with the psychologist and refuse to go back there: they are convinced that Jeremy has a physical illness – not a 'mental problem'.

The general practitioner agrees to support the family, as they are not keen on referral to another consultant paediatrician. Although they will not see any mental health worker themselves, they reluctantly allow the general practitioner to discuss the situation with the primary mental health worker to see if there are any other useful resources available to support the family. The general practitioner does not argue about whether chronic fatigue syndrome is a physical or mental health problem. She remains optimistic, emphasising that the condition usually improves gradually: she suggests that they should make plans to increase Jeremy's activity over time. However, she warns them not to increase his activity too fast, but suggests an initial goal that Jeremy will begin to get up five minutes earlier each day, keeping a diary of the length of time he spends in bed.

The general practitioner then discusses the situation with the primary mental health worker, who suggests a referral to physiotherapy to help the family with a graded exercise programme for Jeremy. The primary mental health worker also suggests a referral to the community school nurse, who can help build links between family and school and sound out the possibility of a gradual reintroduction into school. The general practitioner discusses these two suggestions with Jeremy and his parents, who agree to let her contact both the physiotherapist and the community school nurse.

Over the next few months, Jeremy (accompanied by one of his parents) sees the physiotherapist weekly and the general practitioner once every three weeks. The community school nurse visits the family at home and establishes contact with Jeremy in school when he starts part-time attendance. She encourages him to drop in to her fortnightly school clinic. The general practitioner meets with the physiotherapist, community school nurse and primary mental health worker at the monthly practice meetings. With the combined support of the general practitioner, physiotherapist and community school nurse, Jeremy and his parents agree on small goals that he will be able to achieve, gradually increasing his level of exercise, regularising his sleep and improving his attendance at school. This is monitored through Jeremy's diary. Initial school attendance is erratic; there are a number of setbacks with both the exercise increases and the school attendance – seemingly related to viral infections. Jeremy and his family are told that these setbacks are to be expected, and that they need to persevere.

Over the course of two years, steady improvements are achieved and eventually maintained, and by the start of his first GCSE year, Jeremy is attending school full-time.

**BOX 29.4** Practice Points for chronic fatigue syndrome/myalgic encephalomyelitis

Look upon it as an organic disease (in the current state of knowledge, a 'don't know' attitude may be safest).

Be optimistic – a large variety of treatment components have been shown to work.

Agree a strategy for gradually improving sleep and gradually increasing activity.

Set small, achievable goals.

Monitor progress in sleep, activity levels and overall functioning.

Predict relapse and discuss how to deal with it.

Advise the young person and family not to push too fast for improvements.

Consider and if possible help with associated issues.

## REFERENCES

1  We are indebted to Dr Nigel Speight, retired Consultant Paediatrician, Durham, for adding a fresh perspective to this chapter.

2  Bould H, Lewis G, Emond A, *et al*. Depression and anxiety in children with CFS/ME: cause or effect? *Arch Dis Child*. 2011; **96**(3): 211–14. Epub 2010 Jul 26.

3  Knoop H, Stulemeijer M, de Jong LW, *et al*. Efficacy of cognitive behavioral therapy for adolescents with chronic fatigue syndrome: long-term follow-up of a randomized, controlled trial. *Pediatrics*. 2008; **121**(3): e619–22.

4  Royal College of Paediatrics and Child Health. *Evidence Based Guideline for the Management of CFS/ME (Chronic Fatigue Syndrome/Myalgic Encephalopathy) in Children and Young People*. London: RCPCH; 2004.

5  National Institute for Health and Clinical Excellence. *Chronic fatigue syndrome/myalgic encephalomyelitis (or encephalopathy): diagnosis and management of CFS/ME in adults and children* [NICE clinical guideline 53]. London: NICE; 2007.

6  Bould, op. cit.

7  Fukuda K, Straus S, Hickie I, *et al*. The chronic fatigue syndrome: a comprehensive approach to its definition and study. *Ann Intern Med*. 1994; **121**(12): 953–9.

8  Sharpe MC, Archard LC, Banatvala JE, *et al*. A report – chronic fatigue syndrome: guidelines for research. *J R Soc Med*. 1991; **84**(2): 118–21.

9  National Institute for Health and Clinical Excellence, op. cit.

10  Davies S, Crawley E. Chronic fatigue syndrome in children aged 11 years old and younger. *Arch Dis Child*. 2008; **93**(5): 419–21.

11  Lombardi VC, Ruscetti FW, Das Gupta J, *et al*. Detection of an infectious retrovirus, XMRV, in blood cells of patients with chronic fatigue syndrome. *Science*. 2009; **326**(5952): 585–9.

12  Royal College of Paediatrics and Child Health, op. cit.

13  Rangel L, Garralda E, Levin M, *et al*. Personality in adolescents with chronic fatigue syndrome. *Eur Child Adolesc Psychiatry*. 2000; **9**(1): 39–45.

14  Fry AM, Martin M. Cognitive idiosyncrasies among children with the chronic fatigue syndrome: anomalies in self-reported activity levels. *J Psychosom Res*. 1996; **41**(3): 213–23.

15  Brace MJ, Scott SM, McCauley E, *et al*. Family reinforcement of illness behavior: a comparison of adolescents with chronic fatigue syndrome, juvenile arthritis, and healthy controls. *J Dev Behav Pediatr*. 2000; **21**(5): 332–9.

16  Garralda ME, Rangel L. Childhood chronic fatigue syndrome. *Am J Psychiatry*. 2001; **158**(7): 1161.

17  Smith MS, Martin-Herz SP, Womack WM, *et al*. Illness attribution in adolescents with chronic fatigue or migraine. *Pediatrics*. 2003; **111**(4: Pt 1): 376–81.

18  Richards J. Chronic fatigue syndrome in children and adolescents. *Clinical Child Psychology and Psychiatry*. 2000; **5**(1): 31–51.

19  Nigel Speight, personal communication.

20  Reid S, Chalder T, Cleare A, *et al*. Chronic fatigue syndrome. *BMJ*. 2000; **320**: 292–6.

21  Royal College of Paediatrics and Child Health, op. cit.

# Index